The Changing Nature of Pain Complaints over the Lifespan

The Plenum Series in Adult Development and Aging

SERIES EDITOR:
Jack Demick, *Suffolk University, Boston, Massachusetts*

ADULT DEVELOPMENT, THERAPY, AND CULTURE
A Postmodern Synthesis
Gerald D. Young

THE AMERICAN FATHER
Biocultural and Developmental Aspects
Wade C. Mackey

THE CHANGING NATURE OF PAIN COMPLAINTS OVER THE LIFESPAN
Michael R. Thomas and Ranjan Roy

THE DEVELOPMENT OF LOGIC IN ADULTHOOD
Postformal Thought and Its Applications
Jan D. Sinnott

HANDBOOK OF AGING AND MENTAL HEALTH
An Integrative Approach
Edited by Jacob Lomranz

HANDBOOK OF CLINICAL GEROPSYCHOLOGY
Edited by Michel Hersen and Vincent B. Van Hasselt

HANDBOOK OF PAIN AND AGING
Edited by David I. Mostofsky and Jacob Lomranz

HUMAN DEVELOPMENT IN ADULTHOOD
Lewis R. Aiken

PSYCHOLOGICAL TREATMENT OF OLDER ADULTS
An Introductory Text
Edited by Michel Hersen and Vincent B. Van Hasselt

The Changing Nature of Pain Complaints over the Lifespan

Michael R. Thomas and
Ranjan Roy
University of Manitoba
Winnipeg, Manitoba, Canada

Plenum Press • New York and London

Library of Congress Cataloging-in-Publication Data

Thomas, Michael R. (Michael Ray), 1945-
The changing nature of pain complaints over the lifespan / Michael R. Thomas and Ranjan Roy.
p. cm. -- (The Plenum series in adult development and aging)
Includes bibliographical references and index.
ISBN 0-306-45954-X
1. Chronic pain. 2. Pain--Psychological aspects. 3. Pain in old age. 4. Pain in children. I. Roy, R. (Ranjan) II. Title. III. Series.
RB127.T495 1998
616'.0472--dc21 98-41541
CIP

ISBN 0-306-45954-X

A Division of Plenum Publishing Corporation
233 Spring Street, New York, N.Y. 10013

http://www.plenum.com

10 9 8 7 6 5 4 3 2 1

Printed in the United States of America

Preface

This book has evolved over a very long time. The two of us started our collaborative work in chronic pain nearly twenty years ago. In retrospect, our research activities have spanned virtually the entire adult lifespan. It is this realization that led to our thinking about the possibility of a book that would focus on epidemiological and psychosocial aspects of chronic pain problems at various life stages during adulthood. We finally decided to write this book some two years ago.

The book consists of eleven chapters divided into four parts and an epilogue: (1) Introduction to issues of life transition and life events with emphasis on common childhood chronic pain conditions, a foundation chapter; (2) pain issues in early adulthood; (3) pain issues in the middle years; and (4) pain issues in old age.

Chapter 1 provides an overview of life transition theories and then examines two rather common chronic pain conditions: recurrent abdominal pain and headache in children from both epidemiological and psychosocial viewpoints. Part II consists of three chapters on adolescents and young adults. Chapter 2 considers the psychological and familial issues in Juvenile Rheumatoid Arthritis. Chapters 3 and 4 focus on our work with a nonclinical pain population of young adults. Chapter 3 reviews common chronic pain conditions in that population, and Chapter 4 is concerned with the family functioning of this group.

Part III contains three chapters on the middle-age chronic pain population. Chapter 5 deals with the epidemiology of chronic pain during this life stage, Chapter 6 covers the transitional issues during midlife and their relationship to chronic pain, and Chapter 7 examines the pros and cons of family support for chronic pain patients.

Part IV, also containing three chapters, is concerned with the elderly. Chapter 8 addresses the epidemiology of chronic pain in the elderly, Chapter 9 examines the role of psychopathology in chronic pain in the elderly, and Chapter 10 deals with family and social issues. Finally, Chapter 11 gives us an opportunity to indulge in personal views and perspectives.

It is our sincere hope that this book will fill a gap in the literature and provide the reader with an overview of the intricate nature of the relationship between life transitions and chronic pain.

Contents

PART I. INTRODUCTION

PART II. PAIN ISSUES IN ADOLESCENTS AND YOUNG ADULTS

The Changing Nature of Pain Complaints over the Lifespan

PART I

INTRODUCTION

CHAPTER 1

Life Transition Perspective and Chronic Pain

An Overview

Life transition is a simple concept with very complex implications. From birth to death, we go through somewhat predictable physical, psychological, and social transitions at specific periods of our lives. In this book we explore the issues of pain as they are influenced by developmental and psychosocial factors at each of the life transition stages.

At this point a brief review of the different perspectives of life transition issues may be instructive. The combined work of Jung, Erikson, Vaillant, Levinson, and Neugarten cover most of this topic during this century and provide a comprehensive understanding of the key issues of life transition. Taken together, they illuminate and, at the same time, dispel many myths. First and foremost, life transition must be seen as a naturally occurring phenomenon with some universal features, especially in the physiological domain. The second point worthy of note is that the theories under discussion are rooted in the norms and values of the Western world. They exemplify the cultural divergence, for an older adolescent leaving home is a common and indeed an expected occurrence in the Western countries. In countries like India or China, there is no such expectation. These cultural differences are not entirely attributable to the level of industrialization; cultural values and norms appear to transcend industrialization.

For the sake of economy, only an overview of some of the main theories of transition are discussed. Life transition is not an event, but a passage through time. Each stage of transition is naturally accompanied by multidimensional changes. Childhood to adolescence is perhaps the most dramatic, as the status of the child is relinquished in favor of a developing adult status. This phase is often characterized by family tension and *the* parental struggle between their desire to hold onto the child and at same time provide the child with sufficient autonomy to grow into a responsible adult. This situation is further complicated by the child's diminishing ties to the family. This is also the time when children begin to experience physical changes that bestow upon them adult status.

Another transition of almost equal import, especially in the West with its preoccupation for perpetual youthfulness, is the onset of middle age, that is, the transitional phase from young to old. This phase is characterized by personal reevaluation, profound changes in the family structure, and often beginnings of chronic health problems. Children leaving home, the beginnings of potential "empty nest syndrome," new opportunities for many mothers to explore new careers, and increasing caretaking responsibilities for elderly parents and coping with parental deaths are common features. For women onset of menopause and for men declining physical and sexual prowess are some of the common physiological changes that accompany the middle years.

Erikson's (1980) classification of life stages is probably the most widely known. In Erikson's conceptualization, the entire lifespan is composed of eight stages and each stage presents a crisis and a challenge. This crisis is not a threat but a turning point characterized by heightened vulnerability and increased potential. The stages and the struggles associated with them are as follows:

1. Infancy: trust versus mistrust
2. Early childhood: autonomy versus shame, doubt
3. Play age: initiative versus guilt
4. School age: industry versus inferiority
5. Adolescence: identity versus identity confusion
6. Young adulthood: intimacy versus isolation
7. Maturity: generativity versus self-absorption
8. Old age: integrity versus despair, disgust

It is noteworthy that Erikson divided the entire adulthood spectrum into three stages. On the other hand, it is apparent from his writing that he viewed the adulthood stages as critically important. Even in old age, there is opportunity for growth.

In more recent times, Levinson (1977) proposed a model to study life stage issues by dividing the life cycle into five eras. Each stage has its own specific tasks. In his conceptualization, based on a study of men, transition to midlife presented a special hazard and his conclusion was that crisis is inescapable during this transition. In his investigation, this period was one of crisis for 80% of his subjects. His developmental categories comprised three transitional stages: (1) early adult transition; (2) midlife transition; and (3) late-life transition. His focus was adult developmental phases and the above three categories were further subdivided into seven substages. Successful completion of each phase depended in large measure on the choices made by individuals and each transitional phase was generally predictive of crisis and stress that, if present, interfered with the smooth transition to the next stage. It must be stated that Levinson's work was rooted in empirical research, and some of his hypothesis and theories continue to be investigated by contemporary researchers.

In a comprehensive review of the literature, Rosenberg and Farrell (1976) also found that midlife transition is associated with stress and often maladaptive patterns of behavior. This particular life transition stage is especially relevant to any investigation of chronic pain, as this syndrome tends to appear in the early 40s.

In an investigation of life cycle stage and depression, Mirowsky and Ross (1992) found that depression reaches its lowest level at about age 45 and then increases with age. They hypothesized that losses in later life were the major contributory factors in the genesis of depression. E. Murphy (1982) made similar observations of the role of social factors in the genesis of depression in old age.

One purpose of this brief discussion about the life stage issues and the challenges they present involves introducing another critical element, the appearance of multifaceted problems including age-specific pain problems. Family therapists have noted that families often experience distress and loss of family cohesion during transitional phases. Aa an example the marriage itself, which is easily recognized as a major transition and the beginning of a new phase in the lives of two individuals; the birth of a baby would add another level of complexity. Another point of note is that each life stage has its own peculiar set of life events that may or may not be desirable.

One epidemiological study of psychiatric disorder in a gynecological population found that psychiatric morbidity is associated with events such as divorce, separation, and widowhood (Byrne, 1984). In an investigation of 379 women between the ages of 18 and 61, Bankoff (1994) found that female single parents and women without major life roles such as spouse, worker, or student were the most vulnerable group for poor mental health. The roles of a single-parent mother or loss of social roles are generally associated with one or more transitional life events.

Similarly, a study of an adolescent group revealed that exacerbation of introspection, psychological pain, and symptoms are associated with discontinuities in family life, school, and peer relationships (Mechanic, 1983). Fabrega and Miller (1995) postulated that three specific adolescent problems (eating and bodily appearance, psychological identity or selfhood, and social aggression and delinquency) are products of social and cultural changes produced by unrelenting changes linked to the industrial capitalism of the Anglo-American and Western societies. This study is important for the reason that the problems we commonly associate with adolescent transition phase are not only products of a complex interplay between biological, cultural, and social factors, but are also influenced by political realities.

Sweeting (1995), in a study of children between the ages of 7 and 15 years, found that females over this lifespan showed higher levels of morbidity that males. Reversal of the rates of illness was noted from male children to females as they approached early to mid-adolescence. The author hypothesized that increases in physical complaints among females during this period may be related to the decline in their sense of psychological well-being. It is noteworthy that preoccupation with weight in this age group such as anorexia nervosa is clearly a product of altered societal values where "thin is pretty and desirable." The point is that life stage issues cannot be isolated from prevailing cultural beliefs and myths.

Transition to old age may augur retirement and late adolescence may be the beginnings of the children leaving home. Middle years are filled with significant events such as onset of health problems, death of parents, and not infrequently altered family situation. The point about these events associated with life transition is that they appear to have a relationship, albeit a complex one, with the genesis of various kinds of morbidity. In many of the subsequent chapters, life events as they relate to transition and their association with the etiology of chronic pain syndromes will be discussed.

Transition to middle age has received an enormous amount of attention both in academic and popular literature. Transition to old age is not necessarily viewed with optimism, but there is mounting evidence that retirement is welcomed by many and is not necessarily equated with some kind of social death. In short, life transition is a time of opportunity as well as a time for enhanced psychosocial distress. Since much of this book is a discussion of chronic benign pain from adolescence to old age, we shall now briefly discuss the two most common pain problems in childhood. They are recurrent abdominal pain (RAP) and headaches. The discussion will center on the epidemiology and psychosocial considerations including the significance of life events for these two pain conditions.

RECURRENT ABDOMINAL PAIN

Apley (1975) published his classic paper on pediatric recurrent abdominal pain (RAP) in 1958. Since then, there has been a veritable explosion of research and clinical papers on this topic. He reported a prevalence rate of 11%; of these, only 5% had an organic basis for RAP. Environmental stress was identified as a major contributing factor. Children with RAP were anxious, timid, and even more fussy than those without RAP. A recent paper reported that only 5 to 10% of all RAP cases have identifiable organic causes (Scott, 1994), basically supporting Apley's observation.

In a recent article, Lindberg (1994) observed that several of Apley's findings continued to be confirmed. This observation leads inevitably to the conclusion that psychological factors in the etiology of RAP are predominant. In a large-scale study involving 2457 children at the turn of the century in Norway, among other health problems RAP emerged as a significant childhood syndrome (Seip, 1994).

As a result of this study, school physicians were employed for the first time in that country. In a more recent epidemiological study of abdominal migraine involving 549 boys and 534 girls between the ages of 3 and 11 years, RAP was found in 8.4% of all children (Mortimer, Kay, & Jaron, 1993). A Danish study involving 664 children found the frequency rate of 15% for RAP (Lundry, Sandback, & Juul, 1990). A Swedish study with 1333 children found that 47% children presented a variety of symptoms such as headache, chest pain, and abdominal pain, among other symptoms (Alfven, 1993). Specifically RAP was reported by 19.2% of the children. A most intriguing finding supporting Apley's hypothesis of environmental stress was that children living in areas with a high level of immigrants, low income, and other attending social problems were twice as likely to have RAP compared to children from stable neighborhoods (Alfven, 1993).

RAP is a rather heterogeneous syndrome with complex interactions of biopsychosocial factors. Much of the literature on this topic tends to classify its etiology in either/or terms, namely, biological versus psychological. The limitations of this approach are somewhat self-evident and have been addressed by Barr (1983) and Rappaport (1989). Several alternative methods of classification of RAP have emerged. Barr (1983) proposed a tripartite model that differentiates between organic, dysfunctional, and psychogenic bases for this illness. Using this classification approach for determining etiology, Barr (1983) reported finding only 6% with psychogenic, 34% with organic, and 54% of uncertain etiology in a clinical sample of children with RAP. An interesting aspect of this study was that absence of clear organic factors did not inevitably lead to a psychogenic diagnosis. Yet that practice is alive and well. In a recent paper, Scott (1994) reported that 90 to 95% of RAP cases are of psychogenic origin. Another Swedish epidemiological study involving 1333 children also concluded that headaches, RAP, and chest pains often coexist and are often psychosomatic and probably have a central nervous system (CNS) origin. However, a Romanian report provided further support for Barr's proposition that organic factors were critical in the genesis of RAP (Popescu & Hurduc, 1992).

The Primary Forces Model is perhaps the most prevalent model in the literature (Levine & Rappaport, 1984). Combinations of physiological factors such as gastrointestinal motility with environmental circumstances are the underpinnings of this model. The environmental factors can involve nurturance issues, presence of identifiable illness in the family, interactions with siblings, and level of domestic stress and strain (Levine & Rappaport, 1984). Mogilevsky (1996) noted that this model presented serious research limitations. Many of the constructs described in this model did not have standardized assessment instruments available and the number of variables that had to be incorporated into any research design were too many. Yet, as an effort to enlarge the etiologic field and abandon the Descartian duality, this model remains attractive.

FAMILY AND LIFE EVENTS ISSUES

Family issues are of special import in any discussion pertaining to children. This is for the obvious reason that for a child, family remains the center of its existence for a prolonged period of time. This tie and dependency does not begin to truly dissipate until the advent of adolescence, and even then it continues for a few more years. So, in any discussion of the child's social environment, family assumes great significance. Family environment with all its positive and negative attributes must and does affect the child and their pain behaviors. Hence, the focus on family issues in this chapter.

ABDOMINAL PAIN

In seeking an explanation for this condition, McGrath and Unruh (1987) have suggested that psychological and psychiatric as well as familial factors must be considered. Parental mental and physical illnesses, family structure, modeling of pain behaviors, and family and environmental stress can and do contribute to the genesis of RAP.

Life Events and RAP

In considering family stress, a reasonable point of departure is a review of the association between negative life events and the advent of RAP and abdominal pain disorders. Association between life events and morbidity has assumed greater significance since the original work by Holmes and Rahe (1967) mainly because of improved methodology. In the context of children, life events primarily involve family-related issues, and hence the importance in understanding the impact of life events as well as their contribution to the etiology of abdominal pain.

Some of the early studies produced mixed findings. McGrath, Goodman, Firestone, Shipman, and Peters (1983) found no such relationship between life events and pain in a controlled study of children with RAP and pain-free controls. Similar negative findings were reported by Raymer, Weininger, and Hamilton (1984) in their study of children with ulcerative colitis, Crohn's disease, RAP, and pain-free controls.

Positive associations, however, have been reported both by earlier and more recent studies. Crossley (1982) found a positive association between negative life events and increased rate of hospitalization for children with abdominal pain compared to pain-free controls and children hospitalized for appendicitis. Crossley's findings received further affirmation in a study by Hodges, Kline, Barbero, and Flanery (1984). They compared 30 children with RAP with 67 behaviorally disordered children and 42 healthy controls. Data on life events of the previous 12 months were obtained. Parents of these children also completed a schedule of recent events. Results showed that both experimental groups experienced more life events than the healthy controls. An interesting feature distinguishing the RAP and the behaviorally disordered group was that the RAP subjects reported significantly more serious illness and/or hospitalization of the child, serious illness and/or hospitalization of a sibling, serious illness/hospitalization of a parent, death of a grandparent, decreased arguments between parents, death of a close friend, and change in acceptance by peers. Both groups experienced more life events than the healthy group. No significant differences emerged between the three group of parents on life events. All the events but one noted to be of significance were family related. The authors, however, cautioned against drawing firm conclusions without the benefit of replication studies.

Green, Walker, Hickson, and Thompson (1985) also found higher levels of negative life events in a group of adolescents with RAP, chest pain, or headache compared to those attending for routine examination, organic pain, or acute minor illness. They also warned against making any causal link between life events and morbidity.

Robinson, Alverez, and Dodge (1990) compared 40 children with RAP with 41 children attending a dental clinic, 41 healthy controls, and 17 children who had not been tested for RAP but who met all the criteria for RAP. Results showed that RAP subjects experienced more stressful experiences in the previous few months before the onset of pain, stayed away from school more, showed anxiety in various ways, and had parents who reported more symptoms. Robinson's study is important because the authors concluded that events such as parental separation or divorce are "an important trigger factor in susceptible individuals." This conclusion was based on the finding that a significant temporal relationship was found between stressful life events and onset of abdominal pain. It is noteworthy that the events that had the most noxious effect on the children were related to their primary relationships.

Another study compared RAP patients with patients with peptic disease and children with emotional disorders and found that RAP patients reported fewer negative life events than emotionally disturbed children. RAP patients and their mothers in their report of negative life events did not differ from the well group (Walker, Garber, & Greene, 1993). They concluded that negative life events alone were unlikely to cause RAP.

In a prospective study of 197 children with abdominal pain, Walker, Garber, and Green (1994) examined the role of negative life events along with a number of moderating variables 1 year after a clinic visit by the children. Results showed: (1) an association between low social competence at the first clinic visit and subsequent higher levels of negative life events predicting higher levels of somatic complaints at follow-up; (2) among boys in families with high levels of negative life events, those whose mothers were characterized by high levels of somatic symptoms had higher levels of somatic complaints at follow-up; and (3) children whose fathers showed high levels of somatic symptoms showed higher levels of somatic complaints at follow-up regardless of the levels of life events. A critical finding of this study was the buffering role of social competence (peer support) in protecting children against the negative consequences of stressful life events. Academic competence, however, failed to produce a buffering effect. This study is important not only for its breadth, but also because of its prospective design.

That temporal relationships between stressful life events and onset of RAP exist is supported by albeit limited empirical evidence. Despite this evidence, it would be unwise to view negative life events as anything more than one of the contributory factors. Predisposition, unknown organic factors, personality factors, family environment, and illness behavior may all contribute to the genesis of this disorder. Nevertheless, from a clinical point of view it may be perilous to overlook the presence of negative life events, frequently involving separation and loss, in the lives of RAP patients.

FAMILY ISSUES

Any discussion of family matters and pain and illness must, of necessity, include the interrelated issues between role of family dynamics in the etiology and the role of family members in the maintenance of illness behavior.

Family and Etiology of RAP

It can stated, without the fear of serious challenge, that the role of family dynamics in the genesis of RAP are implicated in some complex ways and yet the mechanisms remain unclear. Research that flowed from Minuchin's psychosomatogenic families failed to demonstrate the causal relationship between specific family characteristics and pediatric abdominal pain of uncertain origin (Roy & Frankel, 1995). A most notable problem encountered in any discussion of the significance of family dynamics and other factors in the etiology of RAP is related to the cause-and-effect issue. What is cause and what is effect remains an unanswered question so far as family dynamics in the etiology of RAP is concerned. McGrath and Feldman (1986) arrived at this conclusion years ago and this tangled state of affairs seems to hold true today. Apart from family dynamics, several studies have shown that parents of RAP children tend to suffer from illnesses (often painful). Again, the consensus seems to be that modeling as a mechanism for RAP remains suspect (Lavigne, Schulein, & Hahn, 1986).

Reinforcement of Pain Behavior

Fordyce's (1983) most significant contribution to the psychology of pain is his operant conditioning model which proposed that pain behaviors are maintained and even enhanced by verbal reinforcement by the intimates of the patient. This proposition has been tested with RAP patients and their families and to date has some degree of validation (Dunn-Geier, McGrath, Roucke, & D'Astous, 1986; Sanders, Shepard, Cleghorn, & Woodford, 1994; Walker et al., 1993; Walker & Zemen, 1992). We shall briefly review some of the more recent studies.

Walker and Zeman (1992) reported on parental encouragement of pain behaviors in a group of RAP children. Parents of children with RAP were more inclined to reinforce pain behaviors than parents of children with non-RAP symptoms. Some interesting gender differences also emerged. Mothers were more likely to engage in pain-reinforcement behaviors than fathers, and girls were more likely to be at the receiving end of such behavior than boys. In other words, mothers were more likely to reinforce pain behaviors in their daughters.

In a subsequent study, Walker et al. (1993) compared parental reinforcement behaviors of RAP children, children with psychiatric problems, and well children and found that RAP children perceived greater parental reinforcement of their pain-related symptoms than children with psychiatric disorders and well children. Another interesting aspect of this study was that parents exhibiting and engaging in pain behaviors were more likely to reinforce illness behaviors in their children. A recent study by Sanders and colleagues (1994) demonstrated the efficacy of cognitive–behavioral family intervention compared to standard pediatric care with a group of children with RAP. They found that the cognitive–behavioral family intervention children reported lower levels of pain than the standard pediatric care group, and that application of operant conditioning techniques to encourage nine healthy behaviors was highly predictive of lowered pain reports at posttreatment.

Summary

The omission in this body of literature must be noted. Studies specifically designed to investigate impact of RAP on family functioning are conspicuously missing. Much of the psychological investigations are focused on parental reinforcement of pain behaviors. This is a critical area of investigation. Nevertheless, understanding of pain reinforcement behavior to the exclusion of other family dynamics draws an incomplete picture and often fails to explain underlying reasons for the existence of parental pain-reinforcement behaviors and problems associated with their elimination in treatment. Second, a child's illness is likely to induce significant changes in family functioning and as well as on the normal development of the child. Research is called for in the above areas if we are to have a broad understanding of the developmental issues, both of the individual patients and their families. Minuchin's work made a beginning, but that body of research came to a grinding halt all too soon.

In this next section we turn to headache as another specific example of an early pattern of pain that is present by adolescence. Headache is the most extensively investigated pain problem of childhood and adolescence (Goodman & McGrath, 1991). Before looking at the specifics of some of the findings from epidemiological studies of headache in children and adolescents, limitations to interpretations need to be discussed. The pain literature on headaches in children and adolescents spans a 20-year interval, which means some studies are weak in design and methodology by today's standards. For example, pain is a subjective experience and any data not including self-report, even if the subject is a child or adolescent, will inherently be inaccurate; however, in many instances past studies reported only parental pain ratings. There are also differences in methods of selecting subjects and criteria used for defining headache, so that even when the same age group and questionnaire format are used there can be highly conflicting findings. For example, Deubner (1977) reported the prevalence of headache in adolescent females as 82%, while

Passchier and Orlebeke (1985) found an 11% prevalence for the same age group using the same questionnaire.

In reviewing the headache literature for children and adolescents there appears to emerge some consistency in the prevalence rates. The first important issue to address is that there are actually two prevalence rates to be considered. There is the occurrence of headache of a nonspecific type that includes all diagnostic categories (e.g., migraine, tension, cluster, and mixed etiology). The nonspecific type of headache appears to have a high prevalence rate typically reported to be somewhere between 70 and 80% during a 1-year interval. Waters (1970), using a sample of 963 subjects between the ages of 15 and 34 years, reported across a 1-year time span that 71% of males and 92% of females reported headaches. Similarly, Sillanpaa (1983) reported for a group of 3784 13-year-old adolescents that 82% had reported headaches during the past year, while Deubner (1977) reported 74% of males and 82% of females aged between 10 to 20 years had headaches during the past year ($N = 780$). Most recently, Linet, Stewart, Calentano, Ziegler, and Sprecher (1989), using a sample of 10,169 adolescents and young adults aged 12 to 29 years, reported 55.9% of males and 73.6% of females indicated they had headaches during the past 4 months. Finally, Brattberg (1994), in an epidemiology study of pain in Swedish school children and adolescents ($N = 1245$) ages 8, 11, 13, and 17, reported that 48% had experienced headaches during the past year.

There are a few studies that report headache frequencies in adolescents lower than the typical prevalence rates between 70 and 80%. Sillanpaa (1983b) reported a 12% prevalence rate for the past year ($N = 3784$) in 13-year-old adolescents, and Passchier and Orlebeke (1985) reported a 12% prevalence rate for headache at least once a month in 2286 adolescents 10 to 17 years old. However, in the Passchier and Orlebeke (1985) study, the lower prevalence figure may have been due to the fact that the prevalence interval used was only a month rather than across the past year.

The second prevalence rate for adolescent headaches across a 1-year interval is specifically for the diagnostic classification of migraine headaches. This prevalence rate is typically much lower and has greater variability, falling somewhere in the range between 3 and 20%. Vahlquist (1955) reported a rate of 7.4% for migraine for 1373

16- to 19-year-olds and a 5.9% rate for 792 20- to 29-year-olds. One serious methodological problem with the study is that since a time frame for the recall was not specified, it does not represent a prevalence rate in the current usage of the term. Billie (1962) likewise did not specify a time interval for the recall period and also did not use self-report. The figures reported were for 9059 subjects, 4.6% for the 10- to 12-year-olds and 5.3% for the 13- to 15-year-olds.

In a stronger methodological study, Deubner (1977) reported prevalence rates of migraine headache for the past year for 780 subjects aged 10- to 20-years old as 15.5% for males and 22.1% for females, while Sparks (1978) reported for 12,543 subjects between the ages of 10 and 18 years that 3.3% males and 2.5% females indicated migraines. Sillanpaa (1983b), using a sample of 2921 of 14-year-olds, reported a 10.6% prevalence rate. Last, in a study with 10,169 adolescents and young adults aged 12 to 29 years, Linet et al. (1989) reported a prevalence rate of migraine of 3.8% for males and 6.6% for females across a 4-week time interval.

In summary, among pain prevalence rates in children and adolescents for establishing possible patterns for pain that can be associated with life transition, headache is the most researched pain condition. A number of good epidemiological studies establish prevalence rates during a 1-year interval for nonspecific headaches as somewhere between 70 and 80%. With specific migraine headaches, the prevalence rates across 1 year intervals are less uniformly established in the literature. There is greater variability reported, but most results generally fall between 3 and 20%, with more studies reporting findings in the lower range of figures. Clearly, adolescence is a time of life transition, as was discussed in the earlier section on RAP and life events. There is also evidence that adolescents who experience frequent headache have more daily stress (Brattberg, 1994), such as a mother having pain, not getting enough sleep, loneliness, and fear of being bullied by other students in school. These findings again are highly suggestive that there is a role that life events play during life transition periods that contributes to the development of chronic pain behaviors likely associated with attempts to cope with life difficulties, resulting in the experience of frequent headaches with children and adolescents.

In seeking explanations for headache prevalence rates among

epidemiological pain studies generally, Dworkin, Von Korff, and LeResche (1992) suggest a dynamic ecological model. In such a model there is an interaction between biological psychological, and social factors. Such a model allows for highly varied individual reporting and pain behaviors. Of all the biological factors associated with patterns of headache, there appears to be only one variable that is consistently reported: A gender variable is present, with females reporting higher prevalence rates. This is true for both nonspecific headaches and migraines. Dalsgaard-Nielsen, Enberg-Pedersen, and Holm (1970) have reported that hormonal factors may be present as systematic causes of headaches. However, Brattberg (1994) reported that 75% of females reporting headache reported no correlation between their periods and headache. From the dynamic ecological model, however, a biological factor once operative (such as development of regular hormonal fluctuations) may dissipate but not before patterns are established in pain perception, appraisal, and social reinforcement that persist. Again, the high frequency of headaches and the hormonal changes occurring during the adolescent transition period of puberty are a cooccurrence that is difficult to ascribe to coincidence alone.

PSYCHOLOGICAL ISSUES

Developmentally, as children get older and assessment methods that use self-report of pain become more reliable, there is increasing research on psychological factors associated with pain. Zuckerman, Stevenson, and Bailey (1987) and Goodman and McGrath (1991) each discuss the importance of psychological distress in the epidemiology of pain, especially for recurrent abdominal pain and headaches in pediatric and adolescent populations. Specifically, the most common psychological distress associated with the pain perception of headache in children and adolescents is depression.

According to Stein, Golombek, Marton, and Korenblum (1991), approximately 20% of adolescents experience marked mood dysfunction thought to be related to the physiological, psychological, and social changes associated with this particular stage in life. Chronic pain has even been described by some investigators as a variant of depressive disorders (Blumer & Heilbronn, 1982). Epidemiological studies in adolescent depression suggest high prevalence rates; the U.S. Department of Health and Human Services (1986) reported that 9.5% of patients admitted to state and county mental health facilities (n = 138,000) with the diagnosis of an affective disorder were under the age of 18 years. In summary, recent studies have reported rates of depression within a variety of clinical samples that range between 33 and 54% (Bernstein, 1991; Hagborg, 1992). Stein et al. (1991) further found that older adolescents (i.e., 18-year-olds) are more prone to depression compared to younger adolescents (i.e., 16-year-olds) and that their depression is thought to be associated with greater levels of stress experienced at that point in life. These findings regarding adolescents and the high correlation between chronic headache pain and reported depression demonstrate that later patterns of depression and chronic pain in clinical populations during adulthood are probably well established before later onset.

Again, a dynamic ecological model of pain (which is one of the most interactive and inclusive models) suggests that common psychological and behavioral dysfunctions such as depression, anxiety, and irritability will develop independent of pain location (such as headache) due to effects beyond the biological etiology. In other words, children and adolescents with chronic headaches that involve dysfunctional behavior probably also come to share common psychological and social characteristics related to life transitions. Dworkin et al. (1992) argue that chronic pain regardless of location shares common psychological mechanisms of pain perception and appraisal and that these in turn reflect the changing cognitive skills associated with transition from child to adult thinking (Piaget, 1972).

FAMILY ISSUES

Clinicians have suggested that many types of pain problems aggregate or cluster in families (Apley & Hale, 1973; Goodman & McGrath, 1991; Thomas, 1994). The family is the focus of several studies looking at headache in children and adolescents (Roy, Thomas Mogilevsky, & Cook, 1994). For this age group the family of origin and the current family are typically the same. Several mechanisms are hypothesized as occurring in families that likely impact on headache reporting in children and adolescents. These include learning generic dysfunctional responses to pain, learning specific dysfunctional responses to headache, modeling of social roles (sick role), and behavioral contingencies.

Children develop pain behavior patterns early in life, which is consistent with the fact that childhood is a period of intense multidimensional life transitions. What is not clear is how family factors interact specifically with life events related to life transition that lead some children into deficient coping skills such that emotional issues become expressed through reports of chronic headaches (Edwards, Zeichner, Kuczmierczyk, & Boczkowski, 1985). The literature that exists, which is very limited, suggests that children from families where chronic pain is present tend to develop pain problems themselves; this is especially the case when the chronic pain is headache (Apley, 1975; Craig, 1978; Violon, 1984, 1985). Chronic pain, which often has a very simple beginning such as a minor trauma, over time becomes a complex epiphenomenon incorporating the biological, psychological, and social aspects established during adolescence. If one were to speculate, the common factor among chronic headache, life events, and periods of life transition is simply change.

SUMMARY

Overall, the developmental roots of attitudes toward pain and illness remain largely indeterminate. The influence of modeling, vicarious conditioning, and personality correlates on pain and illness behavior have been studied primarily in clinical populations (Gentry, Shows, & Thomas, 1974; Ziesat, 1978; Turkat, 1982; Turkat, Guise, & Carter, 1983; Violon & Giurgea, 1984). One useful model for predicting influential mediating variables of health attitudes and behavior for both clinical and nonclinical populations is using life events as a way to help organize understanding pain across the lifespan. This approach uses age as a measure of time to study risk factors and disease presentation through human development.

The focus of this chapter has been on the time span of childhood and adolescence. Already at this early age of development, chronic pain patterns appear in epidemiological studies in the locations of recurrent abdominal pain and headache. Looking at pain across time allows data involving age effects such as pain prevalence associated with aging or cohort effects to become evident. The epidemiological and clinical pain literature clearly show that chronic pain conditions in both populations and individuals vary over time (McGrath & Unruh, 1987; Harkins, 1988). However, there is little systematic evidence regarding how pain varies across different stages of human development. The concept of life transitions in relation to RAP and headaches allows one to see the different patterns between biology, psychology, and social context between childhood, adolescence, and young adulthood. Headache and RAP are conceptualized more often though biological factors and social context rather than psychological factors. This phenomena may reflect in part the fact that there are extremely few reliable ways to assess psychological features associated with headache and stomach pain in children. Not only are there powerful life transition forces acting upon children, but the rapid changes occurring are easier to describe physically and socially through external evaluation when they involve pain. In contrast, psychological introspection, which subjective interpretive pain self-reporting requires, varies tremendously depending on the child's cognitive development, which is undergoing continuous development.

PART II

PAIN ISSUES IN ADOLESCENTS AND YOUNG ADULTS

CHAPTER 2

Coping with Chronic Pain during Adolescence

Juvenile Rheumatoid Arthritis (JRA) in Perspective

Adolescence, a time of physical, social, and emotional transition, by definition is a period of heightened vulnerability. The central preoccupation in the developmental literature on adolescents is fixated on the struggle around identity formation–transition from child to adult, from girl or boy to woman or man. Health-related problems are capable of generating enormous psychic as well as interpersonal conflict in an adolescent. The need to conform and to be acceptable to peers is at its peak during this phase. Any threat to this developing sense of selfhood can pose challenges of extraordinary proportion to an already fragile individual.

Erikson (1980), in his discussion of the adolescent life stage, observed that

> Youth after youth, bewildered by some assumed role, a role forced on him by the inexorable standardization of American adolescence, runs away in one form or another; leaving school and jobs, staying out all night, or withdrawing into bizarre and inaccessible moods. (p. 97)

The poignancy of this observation is that this "forced role" is further challenged and made more complex if the child is in the throes of a chronic and potentially disabling illness. Adolescence is a time for the emergence of sexual identity. The emergence or presence of a chronic disease poses a further threat to the very process of successful completion of this life stage and the emergence into healthy adulthood. Chronic illness in a child has serious ramifications for the family, school, and social environment.

Some years ago, Mitchell (1975) succinctly summarized Cantril's (1964) observations about the human requirement as applied to adolescents. The central purpose for summarizing Cantril's observations is to further emphasize that illness during adolescence poses a qualitatively different challenge than perhaps at any other stage of human development. We shall directly quote Mitchell (1975) to avoid any misinterpretation:

> (1) The adolescent wants security in both its physical and its psychological meaning to protect gains already made and to assure a beachhead from which further advances may be staged; (2) The adolescent craves sufficient order and certainty in his life to enable him to judge with fair accuracy what will or what will not occur if he does or does not act in certain ways; (3) Adolescents continuously seek to enlarge the range and enrich the quality of their satisfactions; (4) Adolescents are creatures of hope and are not genetically designed to resign themselves; (5) Adolescents have the capacity to make choices and the desire to exercise this capacity; (6) Adolescents require the freedom to exercise the choices they are making; (7) Adolescents want to experience their own identity and integrity; (8) Adolescents want to experience a sense of their own worth; (9) Adolescents seek some value or system of beliefs to which they can commit themselves; and (10) Adolescents want a sense of surety and confidence that the society of which they are a part holds out a fair degree of hope that their aspirations will be fulfilled. (p. 224)

A close examination of the needs and aspirations of the adolescent, as outlined above, reveals the depth to which their sense of who they are, their place in society, and their future goals and aspirations are placed in jeopardy in the face of a chronic illness. In developmental terms they are often caught between their emerging autonomy and the inevitable dependency needs created by the illness, thus further exacerbating interpersonal conflict. The greatest impact of this conflict is often felt by the parents.

This chapter purports to explore the key aspects of chronic pain in adolescents first through a general discussion of the impact of chronic illness in an adolescent child on the family, and the child her/himself. Second, the epidemiology of juvenile rheumatoid arthritis (JRA) will be briefly discussed, followed by the individual and family consequences of this disorder.

IMPACT OF CHRONIC ILLNESS IN AN ADOLESCENT ON THE FAMILY

The chronic illness literature pertaining to the adolescent is voluminous. Thus, only some of the more general observations noted in recent literature will be reported. In a recent editorial, Eiser and Berrenberg (1995) made the following observations. Recognizing that diagnosis of a chronic disorder in an adolescent poses major challenges for the parents and their children, they noted that the theoretical explanations or models to explain various family-related phenomena were basically inadequate.

Psychoanalytic models that tended to be prevalent in clinical settings generally lacked empirical validation. Furthermore, the notion that adolescence was inevitably a time of distress and tension, perpetuated by the psychiatric clinical models of the 1950s and 1960s, also lacked empirical validation. These models presumed conflict and tension as necessary accompaniments of adolescence. On the other hand, sociorelational models emphasized the inherent stability of close relationships. These models emphasized continuity rather than change. While at a theoretical level this approach is appealing, Eiser and Berrenberg (1995) found very little work that has investigated the impact of chronic disease on parent–child relationships in any thoroughly systematic and empirically sound way. This will be borne out in the context of JRA and family issues.

Eiser and Berrenberg identified five methodological shortcomings in research on the impact of chronic illness of children on parents. One major source of these shortcomings is the assumption that parental overprotection lies at the heart of this problem. The methodological problems are as follows: (1) Lack of concordance between the responses of parents and children. Questionnaires must be so written to ensure that parents and children interpret the questions the same way. (2) Samples are almost inevitably drawn from clinical populations. In addition, the study population tends to be between the ages of 8 and 21. This creates a serious problem in identifying the developmental issues that tend to vary substantially among the age groups. These factors must be taken into account. (3) As a direct consequence of the disease, pubertal growth can be retarded or even halted. The implications of this factor for family relationships often go unrecognized. Attention should be paid to something as obvious as developmental arrest due to disease. (4) Issues such as "conflict" emanating from parental overprotection have been overemphasized in the literature, whereas the same behavior is interpreted as "monitoring" in the parents of healthy adolescents. (5) Peer relationship among chronically ill adolescents are often seen as obstructive, which is not necessarily so.

Yet, a relatively respectable body of literature exploring the family issues of ill children from a systemic perspective exists. In their comprehensive review of that literature, Roy and Frankel (1995) also arrived at a similar conclusion to Eiser and Berrenberg (1995), namely, that methodologically sound studies were few and far between. Yet, Patterson (1991), citing studies of varying methodological soundness, made a strong plea for the adoption of the systemic perspective for working with youths with disability. In her extensive review of the literature, the quality of studies she chose to report were inevitably presented as acceptable. From a theoretical point of view, the systemic perspective, which attempts to delineate the interconnections and avoid linear relationships, is appealing. It is not just the child's behavior toward the parents but their behavior toward the child that determines their mutual relationship. For a host of methodological reasons, research to demonstrate such an interplay of relationships and their consequences remains in its infancy. Outcome studies of family therapy based on systemic principles with medically ill or disabled persons are sparse and methodologically wanting.

It is against this background that the family issues of JRA must be investigated. First we present a brief summary of the literature on the epidemiology of JRA.

EPIDEMIOLOGY OF JRA

This is a large topic and as such beyond the scope of this chapter. The main purpose of this section is to acquaint the reader with the scope of the problem in terms of its incidence and prevalence. It should also be acknowledged that even with these constraints, the amount of recent work remains significant. Literature is also international in scope, from Kuwait and Turkey to Australia, the United States, Canada, the Caribbean, Britain, France, Germany, Sweden, Belgium, and so on. Reasons for this global interest become self-evident when the scope of the disease and its deleterious effects are fully appreciated. Also, a great many of these studies investigate juvenile chronic arthritis (JCA), which includes JRA. We shall briefly report the incidence and prevalence of JRA and JCA separately.

JRA

Peterson and associates (1996) conducted a retrospective study to investigate trends in the incidence and prevalence of JRA over 33 (1960–1993) years. They screened medical records from 1978 to 1993 for all Rochester, MN residents with a history of JRA, and combined that data set with their own database of JRA from 1960 to 1979. Of 1240 medical records reviewed, 65 cases of JRA were screened between 1960 and 1993. The overall incidence rate per 100,000 population was 11.7. Incidence (shown in brackets) seemed to decline over three discreet periods of between 1960 and 1969 (15.0), 1970 and 1979 (14.1), and 1980 and 1993 (7.8). The authors speculated that environmental factors may indeed influence incidence of this disease.

In a methodologically similar (data collected from existing registries) study where the data for JRA were derived from a disease registry of a local children's hospital in Winnipeg, Manitoba, the incidence rate for JRA between 1975 and 1992 was estimated at 5.34 per 100,000 population (Oen, Fast, & Postl, 1995). Some peaks in the incidence were apparent in 1979, 1982, 1986, and 1990–1991. This study, which attempted to seek correlations between cyclic infections and JRA, raised the possibility of an infectious etiology for JRA. It is noteworthy that the incidence rate in the Manitoba study is 50% less compared to the previous study. The extent to which this differential could be explained by methodological differences, despite similar methods employed for sample selection, remains an important question.

In an earlier, 1-year prospective study of Finnish schoolchildren under the age of 16, the incidence of JRA per 100,000 population was established at 19.6 (Kunnamo, Kallio, & Pelkonen, 1986). A somewhat comparable rate of incidence for JRA—23.6 per 100,000—was found among Inuits of the Canadian High Arctic (Oen, Postl, Chalmers, Ling, et al., 1986). In contrast, the incidence was found to be 6.6 per 100,000 in an urban black population in the United States (Hochberg, Linet, & Sills, 1983).

JCA

A report in 1983 estimated that the prevalence of JCA in the United States was 0.5 cases per 1,000 children or 50 per 100,000; based on 1980 census data, 32,000 children suffered from JCA (Gewanter, Roghmann, & Barin, 1983). A Swedish epidemiological study conducted in 1983 also found a prevalence rate of 56 per 100,000 children in western Sweden. The peak age of onset was 0 to 4 years, and girls predominated over boys in a ratio of 3:2 (Andersson, Fasth, Andersson, Berglund, 1987). A Scottish study also reported a prevalence rate of 2.0 per 1000 for children aged 15 years or younger (Steven, 1992).

A Swedish study reported an average annual incidence of 6.4 per 100,000 in boys aged 12 to 15 years (Gare & Fasth, 1992). In a major study of an urban Belgian adolescent student population of children between the ages of 12 and 18, a prevalence of 167 per 100,000 for definite JCA and 301 per 100,000 for possible JCA was found (Mielants, Veys, Maertens, Goemaere, 1994). In contrast, an Australian study of children 12 and under reported a prevalence rate of 4.0 per 1000 or 40 per 100,000 (Manners & Diepeveen, 1996).

This brief incursion into the epidemiological literature was meant to show the great variation in the estimated rate of incidence and prevalence for JCA. For example, the estimate of children with JCA ranges from 60,000 to 250,000 in the United States (Jaworski, 1993). As was noted earlier, any effort to draw general conclusions are impractical and perhaps of little use because of the sheer variability in design and population under study in these investigations. Yet, the numbers do manage to convey, albeit somewhat erratically, the magnitude of this problem. For the children with this affliction and their families, the breadth and depth of psychological, familial, and general psychosocial problems can be substantial.

PSYCHOPATHOLOGY AND PSYCHOSOCIAL PROBLEMS

As an introduction to the psychosocial and other related matters, we narrate the case of a 21-year-old patient with RA. It must be acknowledged that this patient, by all definition, is an adult. Yet, she contracted the disease as an adolescent and some of the conflicts of adolescence are all too clearly visible in this patient.

A Case of JRA

The case of Gloria encapsulates many of critical psychosocial issues that will be presently reviewed. Gloria, aged 21, was diagnosed with JRA in her teens. She was referred to the authors' pain clinic by her family physician for an investigation of her general mood. The referring physician was very concerned that for Gloria coming to terms with her disease was posing a major challenge. Although this patient was no longer an adolescent, we chose to discuss her situation because many of the common concerns expressed by older adolescents were embedded in this case.

The poignant aspects of Gloria's story were as follows. She married a year earlier, which happened to coincide with a rather unexpected deterioration of her disease. She resisted visiting her rheumatologist for several months. In the meantime, she was finding her job in an animal center rather taxing. Just prior to her arrival at the pain clinic, she received a mild reprimand, and then a week later she was unceremoniously dismissed from her job. This job, which entailed looking after animals, was more a vocation than a job. She had always owned horses, enjoyed riding, and spent an extraordinary amount of time caring for them. She was not a very promising student, just managing to complete grade 12, and had her mind set on getting into a horse-related business, perhaps operating a riding school. Her dream came to a somewhat abrupt end.

She came from a well-to-do family and was the younger of two siblings; her brother was now a successful businessman. Her father was a retired professional and her mother a homemaker. Her family members did not find it easy to discuss her health. Gloria's husband was very understanding and sympathetic. Nevertheless, Gloria's main problem was herself and her almost complete unwillingness, perhaps even inability, to begin to accept the reality of coping with what was potentially a debilitating disease.

Her sense of loss was enormous. In a very real sense, she felt robbed of her one and only dream: to raise horses. To counter her increasing aches and pain, she redoubled her effort to undertake more physical work. She and her husband moved into a new home and this gave Gloria a fresh reason to be physically active.

Visits to her rheumatologist began to assume great importance. Her sense of well-being was severely tested any time her blood tests showed any sign of increase in disease activity. She began to make mental notes of her subjective feelings and increased disease activity, failing to find any direct relationship. This caused her to feel even more frustrated, as her personal feelings of well-being were now and again contraindicated by the level of her disease. She could not always trust her own judgment about how well or ill she was.

Over time, Gloria began to express with great clarity her fears and concerns. Not many of her relatives had any understanding of her diseases. Some were even critical about her job loss, thus compounding her already deflated self-image. Even her parents lacked understanding. Only her husband understood. She began to distance herself from her immediate family. In therapy, she vacillated between an acceptance of the facts that surrounded her disease—that it had an unpredictable course, that she was responding reasonably well to treatment, and her almost total reluctance to consider her options—and the challenging task of redefining herself as someone whose physical abilities were beginning to be compromised.

This redefinition of self, when the sense of self is an adolescent or young adult is still emerging, is most torturous. It is not a simple matter of finding another job or perhaps not working; rather, it is the loss of something profound: Loss of physical prowess, living with at times severe pain, loss of activities, increased dependency and conflict around it, sadness, anger, even depression, temptation to give up, or acting out are all part of this struggle. This struggle depicts the conflict of being forced to give up something familiar and valued for something unknown. Gloria put it this way: "Everything I ever wanted to do does not seem possible any more. Now I have no idea who I am." Erikson's concept of crisis of identity is apparent in that rather sad statement. Gloria's story creates a background for the relevant psychosocial literature that follows.

JRA and Psychopathology

It is a matter of some curiosity that the quantity and quality of literature on this topic are somewhat wanting. The actual amount of attention given to this topic is rather limited. Much of the literature is given to older subjects and varied diagnostic groups. There is some suggestion of enhanced anxiety and depression in this population, some difficulties in coping, and more family problems and increased negative life events.

Hagglund (1995) failed to find any association between pain and a variety of social and psychological factors. On the other hand, level of pain was correlated with duration of disease and age. Children tended to report more pain as they grew but curiously less pain the longer they had JRA. They noted that recently diagnosed children were more likely to report more pain. An interesting finding of this study was the failure of psychological factors including depression to predict levels of pain.

In contrast, a Finnish study found a high rate of prevalence of psychopathology in a group of 54 children with JRA. Two interesting findings were worthy of note: (1) There was a lack of consistency in the personality profile of these children, meaning from a personality point of view the group was heterogeneous; and (2) onset of the disease in a striking 37% of the children was preceded by stressful life events.

This study confirmed an earlier study in the United Kingdom where 80 subjects with RA ranging in age from 18 to 78 years were investigated for psychiatric disorders (Creed, Murphy, & Jayson, 1990). Social stress was a major contributor to psychiatric morbidity in these patients. Based on two separate measures the rate of prevalence was 21% and 24%. The authors warned that symptoms directly attributable to RA may inflate the estimated prevalence and erroneously indicate a direct relationship between the severity of RA and psychiatric morbidity. Vandvik (1990) reported an even higher rate of psychiatric and psychosocial morbidity. Positive psychiatric diagnosis was made in 50% of a group of 98 children recently diagnosed with arthritic disorders. Psychosocial problems of mild severity were evident in 64% of the children.

King and Hanson (1986) noted that children with JRA did not have unique personality characteristics and provided little evidence of social maladjustment. The precise role played by social stress in the onset or exacerbation of the disease remained unclear.

In their review of the impact of JRA on the family, Quirk and Young (1990) concluded that the research findings on this topic were often contradictory. They offered three reasons for this state of affairs: (1) The use of retrospective research designs that do not systematically control for a number of important variables such as duration since diagnosis of the illness, age of the child, and developmental state of adaptation; (2) inadequate sampling techniques; and (3) failure to study the interrelationships among physical signs and symptoms and psychological and interpersonal functioning.

FAMILY ISSUES

Family issues can be divided broadly into three categories: (1) The etiologic significance of family dynamics; (2) the impact of the disease on the various aspects of family functioning; and (3) family treatment issues. It can be stated without fear of contradiction that the role of the family dynamics in the etiology of JRA is unknown. The second aspect is the main focus of this section. The final aspect of family intervention will be briefly reviewed.

Family's Role and Function and JRA

Before we review the pertinent literature, it may be instructive to return to Gloria's case for a brief discussion of relevant family issues. Gloria's parents were not seen by us, but she and her husband John were seen together as a part of a routine psychosocial assessment. As noted earlier, the marriage appeared to be based on a solid foundation. John had taken considerable trouble to make himself knowledgeable about her disease. In a relatively short time, he adjusted to the vagaries of the disease in that he was able to take over family chores when Gloria was unwell. Their sexual relationship was good, though Gloria's level of pain was always a factor. In spite of his considerate attitude toward her, he was never unduly protective of Gloria. He relied on Gloria's judgment to determine her level of activity on a given day.

The situation, however, was vastly different with her parents and relatives. Her father was overly concerned and her mother was preoccupied with her own problems. Some of Gloria's close relatives were dismissive of her condition and were, in fact, incredulous about her level of disability. Gloria tried to resolve these matters by distancing herself from her intimates.

In summary, other than her husband, few members of her family showed much understanding her dilemma, let alone being a source of support and understanding. Parental support could be a key factor in coping with the disease. This lack of support was a factor contributing to Gloria's level of distress, who was in serious conflict about coming to terms with her condition.

One of the factors that impinges on the capacity of the parents to be helpful is their own health and level of social stressors in their lives. Several studies attest to this observation. Vandvik and Forseth (1994), in a study of ten adolescents with fibromyalgia, seven of the mothers and three of the fathers had chronic disorders. High parental expectation was evident in eight families. In an earlier study, Vandvik, Hoyeraal, and Fagurtun (1989) reported high prevalence of family difficulties and recent stressful life events in a study of 116 families of children with JRA. A surprising 75% of the families were faced with chronic family difficulties. The authors regretted the absence of longitudinal studies to assess the long-term impact of the chronic difficulties on the outcome of JRA.

In another study of JRA patients, a strong relationship was found between the level of emotional distress of the mother and level of the child's pain. A somewhat paradoxical finding was that higher levels of family harmony also showed a positive correlation with level of reported pain (Ross, Lavigne, Hayford, Berry, et al., 1993). The precise implication of this last finding is not self-evident.

Nevertheless, there is evidence to the contrary showing that family harmony is an asset rather than a negative force, and at times responses are reciprocal. In a study of 25 young subjects with JRA,

Chaney and Peterson (1989) concluded that effective family functioning led to compliance with self-medication. Yet, family functioning was not related to regimen knowledge or disease activity. A study by Wallander and Varni (1989) also showed the value of family resources in the psychological adaptation of 153 chronically ill children, including children with JRA. Their central finding was that variation in the psychological well-being of the children was related both to psychological and utilitarian family resources. Furthermore, psychological family resources contributed significantly to the prediction of adjustment beyond that provided by utilitarian family resources. In other words, the family as a whole played a major role in determining the adjustment of the children to chronic illness.

Timko, Stovel, and Moos (1992) tested a stress and coping model in which parental functioning was affected by ongoing life stressors, family resources, and parents' illness-related coping. To test their model, they explored the adaptation of mothers and fathers of children with JRA. The sample comprised 159 married couples; 111 of these couples were followed up for a year.

A key finding was that poorer concurrent functioning among both parents was explained partly by patients having more functional disability, pain, and psychosocial problems. The reciprocal aspect of this finding is critical to understanding the essence of the systemic dynamics of family functioning. Change in any part of a given system will influence all related subsystems. Mothers reported both more depression and mastery, but both parents were similar in terms of stress and coping factors that determined their levels of functioning. However, it is noteworthy that both parents had considerably lower scores compared to a group of clinically depressed adults. More family resources were related to less depression.

The authors concluded that the main findings of this complex study had implications for intervention. Since similar types of risk factors were involved in both parents' functioning, common interventions could be helpful to both parents. The goal of such an intervention would be to help parents improve their functioning in the disrupted areas. Otherwise, the problems are likely to continue.

A literature review by Ross and associates (1993) concluded that a variety of family, parental, and child variables influenced child and sibling adaptation to JRA. Despite serious methodological deficiencies, new advances were facilitating improved understanding of children and adolescents with JRA. In his review of the psychosocial literature pertaining to JRA, Jaworski (1993) noted that in recent years significantly improved methodologies have been employed by researchers in this field. Longitudinal studies were called for to investigate lasting or long-term effects of family factors on JRA. This body of literature tends to confirm a generally held belief that the family plays an intricate role in JRA. The family impacts on the child and vice versa. Families with resilience, those who adapt to the changing demands of living with a young person with JRA, those who show psychological family resources, or families that are "healthy" are best suited to provide a nurturing environment and enable their children to cope successfully with their disease. The centrality of the family in the treatment of JRA is well illustrated by the group of studies we discussed above.

Social Support and JRA

Social support has emerged as a major area of investigation over the past few decades. The theory underlying the concept is that effective social support acts as a buffer against morbidity, or in the presence of morbidity its effects are modified. A limited body of literature in relation to arthritic diseases in juveniles and mixed age groups now exists that tends to confirm the usefulness of effective social support (Doeglas et al., 1994; Revenson, Schiaffino, Maljerovitz, & Gibofsky, 1991; Timko, Stovel, & Baumgartner, 1995; Varni, Wilcox, & Hanson, 1988; Wallander & Varni, 1989). Three of these studies are related to children and clearly show the benefits of social support (Timko et al., 1995; Varni et al., 1988; Wallander & Varni, 1989). However, there is also some evidence to the contrary, where the value of social support is not evident (Hagglund et al., 1995). A brief discussion of the key findings of these studies follows. It should also be noted that social support is intricately related to family support.

Varni and associates (1988) explored the mediating power of social support on psychological adjustment in 23 subjects aged 5 to 15 years with JRA. Family social support was found to be a significant predictor of psychological adjustment, accounting for 22% of variance in each of the areas of internalizing and externalizing behavior problems. The importance of family support received endorsement in this study.

Wallander and Varni (1989) confirmed the above finding. In addition, however, they found that peer support in conjunction with family support contributed to significantly better adjustment than high social support from any one of the two sources alone.

In a study of 94 adolescents aged 12 to 23 years with JRA, Timko and colleagues (1995) examined the relationship between acute and chronic life stressors, stable social resources, and psychosocial functioning. Their key finding was that despite a lack of any association between life stressors and social resources to disease outcomes, subjects who experienced more acute negative events and chronic life stressors and who lacked stable social resources showed worse psychosocial functioning. From the view of family support, family resources moderated the relation of acute and chronic life stressors to psychosocial functioning.

The significance of these three studies is that (one way or another) they confirmed the value of family support as well as family resources in moderating the negative effects of the disease or in exerting a protective barrier to psychosocial problems. The value of the family as a major, if not the main, support system in these studies lends further credence to the adoption of a family-oriented approach in the overall treatment of JRA. Yet, as the following section reveals, family intervention, at least as reported in the literature, remains an underutilized therapy.

Family Intervention

Generally, the use of family therapy has not found much favor with the medically ill and their families. A recent comprehensive review of the literature showed that while clinical application of this method of treatment has been extensively reported in the literature, there is a remarkable absence of any outcome studies (Roy & Frankel, 1995).

Despite clear empirical evidence that families affected by JRA encounter a variety of problems, the family therapy literature is conspicuous by its absence. A careful literature search failed to demonstrate research using family therapy. Finney and Bonner (1992) conducted a review of the family therapy literature, especially behavioral family interventions designed to treat a variety of medical conditions including JRA, and concluded that behavioral oriented family therapy had not been rigorously evaluated for its efficacy. These authors did indicate, however, optimism for systems-based family therapy approach with medical conditions. The virtual absence of family therapy outcome studies for JRA is a serious omission in the literature. Yet, it is possible that health care practitioners do employ family therapy as an adjunct treatment with this group of patients and their families. There is limited evidence to support this belief. A University of Minnesota survey of the activities of family therapists showed that physical illness was indeed one of the presenting problems that family therapists encountered with some degree of frequency (Simmons & Doherty, 1995). Another investigation of the referral patterns of a child psychiatry liaison service revealed that reasons for referral were management of physical illness or nonorganic physical complaints. Furthermore, a frequent diagnosis was of "anomalous family situation," and the main intervention was family therapy (McFayden, Broster, & Black, 1995). However, literature on the entire topic of family therapy with adolescent physically ill patients and their families is virtually nonexistent. The general family therapy literature on the problems of adolescence is voluminous but mostly pertains to psychiatric conditions.

In the absence of pertinent literature, a summary of brief family therapy with a 16-year-old patient, Joan, an only child, with JRA and her parents is presented. This patient was referred to one of the authors for her noncompliance with the treatment regimen. She was a model inpatient, but once she returned home, there were drastic changes in her behavior. She would party till late hours, often engage in arduous physical activities such as baseball, fail to take her medication, and almost totally ignore her parent's concerns. The parents were beside themselves with worry and in desperate need of help. As a first step, a meeting between the rheumatologist and the family was arranged, during which the physician reinforced the need for compliance, emphasizing that unless Joan listened to her parents and complied with treatment regimen, she would be spending more time in the hospital than was necessary. Need for family intervention was also reinforced, although Joan let it be known that she was in no mood to waste her precious time "talking to a shrink."

This type of resistance is very common in medically ill patients who fail to see any obvious connection between their condition and the need for psychotherapy. In that situation a simple commonsense explanation is called for. In this instance, Joan was asked to consider that life at home was filled with conflict with her parents. She complained constantly of being cramped by them and of course there was no end to their nagging. Would it not be useful if all of them could sit down for a chat to make life a easier for all of them? Joan reflected on this proposition and halfheartedly agreed that she would attend one session to determine if this was not a complete waste of time for her.

In the main, the first session was a catalogue of complaints from Joan. She felt misused by all. The following is a telescoped view of five sessions with this family over a period of 2 months:

> Joan seemed most concerned with being different from her friends. She had to work hard to be like the others, but her mother, according to Joan, was singularly incapable of understanding this fact. Her mother became visibly angered by Joan's outbursts and her father seemed to retreat further into himself. The battle of wills between mother and daughter was very obvious. Father's peripheral role in the family was also apparent. This was a source of great distress for his wife, as she felt—quite correctly—that she had ended up carrying most of the family burden, and to top it all was regarded by Joan as the enemy.
>
> The task of the therapy was to join the parents in common goals and to prescribe homework that would promote joint decision making and common goals and purposes. The other aspect of this intervention was to modify the nature of the struggle between mother and daughter. This had two elements. First, that Joan should be able to engage in some activities that would not jeopardize her health, and second, that her mother would stop being so overprotective. Father's task was to support his wife to achieve this goal. In other words, it was important that Joan saw her parents as working together. To determine what sorts of activities Joan could safely engage in, consultation was sought with physical and occupational therapists, who, along with Joan, worked out a plan. The parents and therapists were to ensure that Joan adhered to the plan. However, the most important aspect of this plan was that Joan herself had to take responsibility for her own actions.
>
> A number of issues are noteworthy. First, Joan's concern about her

identity and her fear of being different from her peers accounted for some of their noncompliance. Mother's overinvolvement and protectiveness, very common and understandable in this situation, contributed to Joan's rebelliousness. Father's peripheral role in the family and his failure to support his wife led Joan to believe that her father was on her side. Therapy resulted in bringing the father into the family orbit and becoming a source of support for his wife and lowering her sense of isolation and anxiety. By having the parents and the health care professionals ensure Joan's adherence to the activities plan, but most of all by making Joan responsible for her own behavior, much of Joan's noncompliance disappeared. The family was seen in long-term follow up, and the changes in the family system seemed to be holding.

A note of caution must be injected at this point. This brief and successful account of family intervention is anecdotal. There is, as yet, a complete absence of outcome studies in family therapy to claim success for this method of intervention with JRA or in counteracting noncompliance through the application of family therapy.

SUMMARY

This chapter has presented JRA as a prototype for chronic pain. The literature on JRA does not always differentiate between younger children and the adolescent population. This made the focus on the adolescent group somewhat diluted. Nevertheless, the problems discussed in this chapter generally confirm that JRA is not an uncommon medical problem. This illness is often associated with complex family problems and related psychosocial issues. The value of effective support systems is reinforced in study after study. Again, the value of the family as a source of support for the patient is reiterated.

CHAPTER 3

Common Chronic Pain Conditions in a Nonclinical Population of Young Adults

The distinction between adolescence and young adulthood is not always clearly delineated in terms of physical and psychological maturity. Thus, in looking at issues of life transition as conceptually related to pain in young adults, there is overlap both with adolescence and middle age. Functioning as a young adult brings with it many first experiences (career and marriage) with new responsibilities and accompanying increased levels of stress. First, this chapter will look at prevalence rates of pain at common locations for individuals across this age interval.

There are a number of nonclinical chronic pain conditions frequently reported in late adolescence through young adulthood. Sternbach (1986a,b) conducted a phone survey on pain complaints that included individuals ranging in age from 18 to 35 years. One conclusion was that younger adults are more likely to experience pains of every type than are older persons, with the exception of joint pains, which increase sharply with age. This reported finding of a general inverse relationship between increasing age and pain complaints with the exception of joint pains has been found by others (Roy & Thomas, 1986, 1987; Thomas & Roy, 1988; Thomas, Roy, & Makarenko, 1989; Mobily, Herr, Clark, & Wallace, 1994), although not universally (Helme & Gibson, 1996).

Chronic pain patients are typically profiled in the research literature as middle-aged individuals in their 40s. In contrast, pain in nonclinical general populations is stereotypically viewed as a problem of the elderly. As a result of these common public perceptions, little interest and research has focused on chronic pain and nonclinical pain in the young adult. What research there is in the pain literature for this age group primarily focuses on unusual illnesses or accident-related trauma. It would appear that the expectations surrounding life events for most young adults typically is focused on establishing careers and lifelong partnerships leading to their own families. However, recent studies in nonclinical populations (Sternbach, 1986a,b; Thomas, Roy, Cook, & Marykuca, 1992) have reported high frequencies (18 to 23%) of self-reported pain in this age group.

Thomas, Roy, and Cook (1992) reported that 23% of a university population had current pain and 10% indicated chronic pain. Demographic studies of pain in general nonclinical populations that included young adults have not systematically looked at the distribution differences in frequency and location of pain with these age groups. However, those pain studies that have looked at young adults all report frequent, intermittent, and even chronic pain (Jack, 1981; Sternbach, 1986; Thomas, 1993; Thomas & Roy, 1995).

Thomas (1993a) reported findings from a 5-year series of studies looking at pain complaints in approximately 1300 young adults (mean age, 19.5 years). Included in this series of studies were pain reports not only from university students but also accompanying pain reports from smaller samples of parents, siblings, and dating partners. Subjects were 1363 first-year university students recruited through introductory psychology courses. Criteria for selection of subgroups of subjects varied. For example, 202 students were selected on the basis that they and their parents both filled out a general health and pain questionnaire to look at family pain patterns. In the next subgroup, 108 were students selected on the basis of having chronic pain that was not responding to current medical treatment. Another 201 students were selected on the basis that they their parents and their long-term dating partners all filled out a health, pain, and sympathy questionnaire. In another subgroup of subjects, 408 students were selected to answer questions about their pain as well as the severity of parental physical punishment during their childhood. In the last subgroup of subjects, there were 222 students and an additional 222 of their closest-aged siblings who filled out a health and pain questionnaire. All subjects, however, answered a core of common questions composed of demographic questions, health history, pain descriptions, depression scores, and self-esteem scores. Different subjects selected by different criteria responded to varied other psychological measures. A demographic profile of this large Canadian student sample based on age, sex, family income, religious affiliation, and employment status indicated that this sample was representative of first-year university students along most social economic status dimensions.

In one of the first investigations conducted in this multigrouped young adult university sample was a comparison between a group that reported chronic clinical pain and a group that reported only intermittent pain. The two groups were compared on their medical histories for common childhood diseases, injuries, and handicaps. In almost all instances the young adults reporting chronic pain also reported higher frequencies of common childhood illnesses and diseases. These findings suggested that a "sick role" was probably already established prior to their current chronic pain experiences. Thus, life transition to young adulthood may impact those individuals with already well-established pain behaviors differently than young adults reporting pain related to stresses of transition in becoming adults.

Next, those subjects with and without chronic pain were compared on most frequent pain locations, severity, duration, and additional collateral information regarding treatment. The chronic pain group reported higher frequencies of pain at all five common pain locations surveyed. As well, the young adults in the chronic pain group also reported higher incidence of collateral pain behaviors such as missing school and taking medication more frequently (see Table 3.1). Of particular interest, however, was the finding that the pain reported by all the young adult subjects from both the chronic pain group as well as the non–chronic pain group tended to be of low severity. There were two exceptions to these reports of frequent but low pain severity. The exceptions to generally low pain severity ratings were headache and back pain in the chronic pain group. These findings of overall low pain severity reported by young

Table 3.1. Student Pain Demographics[a]

	Students from a general university population with current pain (n = 250)	Students from a university population with current chronic pain (n = 108)	
1. Have pain today	30.7%	62%	
2. Pain is due to accident	23.7%	37.1%	
3. Treatment reported helpful	30.7%	38.2%	
4. Taking medication	10.5%	79.6%	
5. Using alcohol to relieve pain	8.7%	16.8%	
6. Pain intensity today Numeric Rating Scale (1–10)	2.8	4.3	
	Students from a general university population who reported past chronic pain (n = 304)	Students from a university population with current chronic pain (n = 108)	
7. Have had past chronic pain	35.7%	100.0%	Duration > 3 months
8. Average duration in months	38.0	51.4	
9. Pain interfered with school	11.4%	48.6%	
10. Treatment of past pain helpful Numeric rating scale (1–10)	6.1	1.8	

[a] n = 840 (missing data ± 15%).

Table 3.2. Average Ratings of Pain Severity by Pain Location[a]

	General student sample (n = 638)	Chronic pain sample (n = 108)
1. Head	2.62	3.03
2. Neck	2.00	2.67
3. Back	2.41	3.31
4. Muscle	2.11	2.53
5. Chest	1.73	2.01
6. Joint	1.94	2.57

[a]Rating scale 1–5: 1, no pain to 5, most severe pain.

adults are consistent with those reported in other studies (Von Korff et al., 1988) (see Table 3.2). In addition, the psychological functioning profile of scores for depression, self-esteem, disability, denial, and somatizating for the chronic pain group did not fall within psychopathological ranges. It would seem that although there was widespread pain reported across a typical week for the subjects in the larger sample of young adults ($N = 1363$) ranging from 30% to 62% depending upon the location (see Tables 3.3–3.5), the pain was minimally disabling due to low levels of severity reported.

Next, Thomas and Roy (1995) conducted a series of regression analyses with the larger composite sample of university students that looked at combinations of demographic, health history, ratings of disability, and psychological functioning as factors associated with

Table 3.3. Illness Behavior Questionnaires (IBQ) Mean Score[a]

	General student sample (n = 522)	Chronic pain sample (n = 108)
1. General hypochondriasis	1.49	1.89 (0–9)[b]
2. Disease conviction	1.27	2.36 (0–6)
3. Psychological vs. somatic	1.87	1.55 (0–4)
4. Affective inhibition	0.97	0.93 (0–5)
5. Affective disturbance	0.86	1.27 (0–5)
6. Denial of life	2.13	1.85 (0–5)
7. Irritability	0.75	1.07 (0–5)

[a]All scores were in the nonclinical range.
[b]Numbers in parentheses are the range.

Table 3.4. Additional Psychological Measures

	General student sample (n = 840)	Chronic pain sample (n = 108)
Beck Depression	8.07	10.18[a]
Rosenberg Self-Esteem Scale	31.54	31.19[b]

[a]Nondepressed.
[b]Normal range.

reported pain locations, severity, duration, and helpfulness of treatment. Of the regressions only one predicting pain duration was strong enough to have practical implications. Pain that was likely to be longer-lasting in a young adult population was associated with higher pain intensity, caused by an accident, were more debilitating socially, and was related to lower self-esteem as well as taking antidepressant medication (Table 3.6).

PREVALENCE BY PAIN LOCATION

Following the Thomas and Roy (1995) study, Thomas (1994) reported detailed information on comparative frequencies for different pain locations during a past-week interval. The sample surveyed

Table 3.5. Student Mean Pain Disability Scores

	General student sample (n = 522)	Chronic pain sample (n = 108)
Questions: How much does pain interfere with your ...?[a]		
1. Family/home duties	1.18	2.56
2. Recreation	1.62	4.28
3. Social activity	1.25	2.41
4. Occupation	1.27	3.18
5. Sexual behavior	0.77	1.53
6. Self care	0.72	1.47
7. Life support activity	0.66	1.43
Total disability score[b]	7.53	16.53

[a]Individual disability question scale range 0–10.
[b]Total disability scale range 0–70.

Table 3.6. Regression Models for Students in Canadian General Population: Variables Predicting Duration of Pain Today

Variables[a]	R^2 partial	R^2 model	Prob > *F* value
1. Pain dis:life supt[a]	0.19	0.19	0.009
2. Rain due accident	0.13	0.33	0.019
3. Self-concept	0.13	0.47	0.009
4. Pain intensity	0.07	0.54	0.037
5. Taken meds depress	0.07	0.61	0.034
6. Pain dis: total sc[b]	0.10	0.72	0.004

[a]Six variables account for 72% of variance (n = 502).
[b]Pain disability scale.

was a young adult sample of university students and their siblings closest in age (N = 444, age range 13 to 25 years old). The university subjects and their siblings were assigned to one of four groups. The first group comprised full biological siblings; the second group comprised identical twins; the third group comprised half siblings; and the fourth group comprised step siblings (Table 3.7). All the young adults in this study reported on pain during the past week at six common locations: (1) headache, (2) neck, (3) back, (4) chest, (5) muscle, and (6) joint. For all groupings, headache, muscle, and back pain were the most frequent locations of reported pain and chest pain was the least frequently reported pain location. This finding was consistent with the previous literature (Crook, Rideout, & Browne, 1984; Thomas, Roy, & Cook, 1992).

Table 3.7. Demographic Data for Sibling Subsample

Variable	Identical twins (n = 18)	Natural siblings (n = 360)	Half siblings (n = 34)	Step sibling (n = 32)
Age	17.9	19.1	19.8	19.2
Males	66.7%	56.6%	55.9%	62.5%
Females	33.3%	43.4%	44.1%	37.5%
Family income	72,000	68,000	67,000	86,000
Average number of siblings	1.8	2.3	2.7	2.1

It would appear that because chest pain was the least common site for pain for these young adults, it generated greater concern when it occurred, since typical pain behaviors indicated that for all subjects chest pain was the pain location rated most likely to prompt a visit to a physician and the location most likely to cause subjects to miss work or school. In contrast, for all subjects, headache was the pain consistently rated as most severe, the pain location most likely to prompt taking medication, and the location that interfered most with social activities and responsibilities (Table 3.8).

The demographics in this sample of students and their siblings strongly suggested that it was a representative sample on several dimensions of Canadian university students between 18 and 25 years old. For example, the ratio of sex of pairs sampled was the same as would be expected from a random population sample (Table 3.9). Prevalence rates for current pain reported in this sample of young adults was 25.3%, which is generally consistent with other studies where current pain ranged between 15% (Jack, 1981), 20% (Crook, Rideout, & Browne, 1984), 18% (Sternbach, 1986a), and 20% (Thomas, Roy, & Makarenko, 1989). Thus, the reported pain frequencies by location in these series of studies continue to contradict the view that normative health in a general sample of young adults is generally pain free.

Table 3.8. Reports of Pain by Location in Past Week in Sample[a]

Pain location	Identical twins (%)	Natural siblings (%)	Half siblings (%)	Step siblings (%)
Headache	72.2	54.1	52.9	71.8
Neck	22.2	23.3	26.4	34.3
Back	33.3	32.2	38.2	46.8
Muscle	44.4	34.7	26.4	34.3
Chest	11.1	9.4	5.8	3.1
Joint	11.1	17.2	23.5	25.0

[a]Percentages are greater than 100% because reports for location were not mutually exclusive.

Table 3.9. Subject Demographics from Intact Families of Twins and Biological Sibling Pairs

Twin pair distribution by sex		
Male/male	6 pairs	67%
Female/female	3 pairs	33%
Biological sibling pair distribution by sex		
Male/female	90 pairs	50%
Male/male	51 pairs	28%
Female/female	39 pairs	22%

FAMILY PATTERNS OF PAIN FOUND IN YOUNG ADULTS

Thomas (1994) found that the distribution of pain complaints in young adults was not random across individuals but instead was focused frequently within some families and not present or minimally so in other families. For example, it was found that both members of sibling pairs within families reported pain in the same location at one of six possible sites with high frequency in the past week (Table 3.10). This result was generally consistent with the clinical pain literature where Payne and Norfleet (1986) reported that 78% of family members of chronic pain patients also reported pain. Apley

Table 3.10. Siblings Pairs Where Both Reported Pain at the Same Location During the Past Week (Only from Subjects Reporting Pain)[a]

Pain location	Identical twin (%)	Biological siblings (%)	Half siblings (%)	Step siblings (%)
Headache	61.5	55.3	33.3	78.2
Neck	50.0	30.9	22.2	36.3
Back	33.3	39.6	46.1	53.3
Muscle	50.0	40.0	22.2	54.5
Chest	00.0	11.7	00.0	00.0
Joint	00.0	16.1	25.0	50.0

[a]Pain locations are greater than 100% because data reports for multiple pain locations across the week interval.

(1975) also found that clinical pain in one sibling was associated with six times the frequency of pain in other siblings compared to controls. Family influences appear to be critical in the distribution of clinical pain behaviors in young adults. Yet, it is still not clear what mechanisms are responsible for a skewed distribution of pain complaints within family units rather than having pain complaints randomly distributed on an individual basis in young adults. These findings suggest that life transition factors operate not only on individuals but families of origin as well with regard to pain features such as location for most frequent pain complaints.

In another study, Thomas, Roy, and Cook (1992) also investigated the distribution of reported pain location within families. This time, however, the investigation looked at similarities in pain locations between young adult university students and their parents as well as their long-term dating partners. Two hundred university students responded to a pain questionnaire on different pain locations. As well as similarities in location of most frequent pain complaints, the subsamples of dating partners and parents (31 dating partners, 37 mothers, and 30 fathers) also provided a validity check on students' reports of location for their pain complaints. Results indicated approximately 23% of the students in this sample reported current pain, with 15% reporting currently taking medication for their pain. Nineteen percent stated they had chronic pain and 21% of these reported being in treatment for their chronic pain. In regard to family patterns for pain location, male students and their fathers tended to complain of back pain most frequently, while female students and their mothers had the greatest similarity in headache complaints.

EXPLANATIONS FOR REPORTED PAIN DISTRIBUTIONS

The pain literature has investigated several possible explanations that could account for biasing factors in distribution of pain complaints in young adults. Possible explanations include such widely divergent transmission mechanisms as reinforcement and modeling to genetic predispositions for the development of pain behaviors (Edwards et al., 1985; Violon & Giurgea, 1983). As can be seen from the most common factors investigated in the pain literature, there is almost no discussion of the role age and life stage may play on changing demographic patterns of pain complaints between young adults and children or middle-aged individuals. There also is no discussion of the impact of life transition on changes in trends for most common pain locations as a function of age.

Attempts to explain systematic patterns of location for pain complaints by age, family, or gender have focused most often on learning theory. This theory asserts that reinforcement patterns of family members for pain behaviors are the primary mechanism to influence individuals' pain complaints (Flor, Turk, & Rudy, 1989). For example, reinforcement of pain behaviors by parents at an early age could influence lifetime pain experiences of individuals (Turk, Flor, & Rudy, 1987), such that parents who positively respond to their children when they express illness behaviors may predispose their children to chronic pain problems in the future (Turkat & Adams, 1982). Vicarious learning by observing family models is another possible explanation that might influence distribution of pain complaints, causing them to be focused within families. This process could also be responsible for transmitting physiological responses, which are associated with the experience of pain, from parents to children (Violon & Giurgea, 1983).

Alternately, the skewed distribution of pain reports within families may indicate the possibility that certain pain experiences are inherited (Edwards et al., 1985). Wolf (1978), for example, through his comparisons of the prevalence of migraine headaches in mothers and their children, asserted that migraine pain is transmitted through a recessive gene. The possibility that individuals inherit vulnerabilities of certain organ systems or "hypersensitivity to nociceptive stimuli" (Turk et al., 1987) that contribute to the occurrence of pain experiences have also been suggested.

Another possible genetic explanation has been that particular physical conditions are inherited, such as lower physical energy levels or excessive sympathetic arousal, which would have implications for the experience of pain (Edwards et al., 1985). In the pain literature, chronic headaches, lower back pain, dental pain, and general pain indicate some possibility of a transmission process of pain complaints in families (Turkat, Kuczmierczyk, & Adams, 1984; Turk et al., 1987). Although most research dealing with the transmission of pain behaviors to younger children and adolescents has focused on clinical populations, these data indicate that the transmission of pain behaviors in non–chronic pain families may also occur, resulting in nonuniform distribution of pain complaints in young adults (Thomas, 1994). Although it might appear that genetic explanations for distribution of pain complaints in families would be incompatible with life transition concepts regarding pain, this is not the case. By their very nature, important life transitions (such as puberty) along some dimensions occur primarily as the result of genetically triggered and determined physical events.

SYMPATHY AND DISTRIBUTION OF PAIN COMPLAINTS

Continuing to look for an explanation for the nonrandom distribution in pain reporting in young adults, Thomas (1993a) investigated sympathy and family constellations. One type of life transition that is becoming a more frequent experience for individuals and families is divorce and remarriage. Patterns of pain complaints from families experiencing divorce and remarriage were compared with families remaining intact. There were four family patterns investigated. Intact families were defined as those with children where one child was a young adult attending university and their sibling was an (1) identical twin or (2) full biological sibling, while blended families were defined as having one child who was a young adult attending university and their sibling was either a (3) half or (4) stepsibling.

Perceived sympathy by family members has been shown to influence pain reporting in clinical populations (Edwards et al., 1985; Romano, Turner, Jensen, Friedman, et al., 1995). Results indicated that mothers were perceived as the most sympathetic family member independent of all pain locations. Fathers were perceived as the next-most sympathetic family member but only in natural biological families (composed of twins and full siblings). In contrast, in the blended families, siblings and fathers were perceived as roughly equal in sympathy across pain locations. Interestingly, parental sympathy for their children's pain appeared highest in biological families as compared to blended families. For blended families with genetically unrelated stepsiblings, perceived sympathy for pain was generally seen as equal when coming from fathers and stepsiblings. Although circumspect, these findings are suggestive that life transition events such as divorce and remarriage indeed do impact on factors influencing pain behaviors in young adults.

To summarize, the highest ratings of perceived sympathy within the family were not systematically related to the most frequently reported pain locations in young adults. As well, the high and consistent ratings of sympathy from mothers toward pain did not necessarily explain the skewed distribution of pain complaints in young adults, since ratings of perceived sympathy were not significantly higher within families where both siblings reported pain as compared to families where only one or even no siblings reported pain. These findings, along with the lack of equivalent levels of frequencies in pain locations between parents and children, suggest that neither sympathy alone nor modeling appear to explain the distribution of pain complaints found in families with young adult siblings. Life transition events in the families of origin appear to be a factor influencing pain in young adults (Table 3.11).

Another theoretical explanation for the apparently nonrandom distribution of pain complaints individually across young adults is genetic. The biological relatedness between siblings has been investigated for the similarity in frequencies and locations of pain complaints. The data reported did not indicate a significant relationship between reported pain locations and the degree of genetic commonality between siblings. In fact, there were indications to the contrary, emphasized by the group of stepsibling pairs who reported similarity for pain locations (with one exception) greater than the pairs of identical twins. However, there was a significant interactive effect between genetic relationship and the environmental factor of time living together in a family setting for similarity in pain complaints in siblings. This finding appears to be consistent with the clinical literature, where it has been reported that clinical pain in one sibling was associated with six times the frequency of pain in other siblings as compared to controls (Apley, 1975). Similarly, Payne and Norfleet (1986) reported 78% of family members of chronic pain patients also reported pain.

Table 3.11. Reported Sources of Sympathy Ratings for Pain Locations

	Father (n = 18)	Mother (n = 18)	Sibling (n = 18)
Twins			
Headache	5.7	11.5	2.9
Neck	6.2	10.4	3.1
Back	6.8	11.7	3.7
Muscle	6.2	10.7	3.7
Chest	5.5	9.4	3.7
Joint	6.6	10.1	3.2
Total	38.1	64.1	20.2
	Father (n = 360)	Mother (n = 360)	Sibling (n = 360)
Biological siblings			
Headache	7.3	11.7	5.9
Neck	7.6	11.6	6.1
Back	8.2	12.4	6.8
Muscle	7.7	11.4	6.2
Chest	7.6	11.2	6.1
Joint	7.2	10.8	6.0
Total	46.3	68.6	37.2
	Father (n = 34)	Mother (n = 34)	Sibling (n = 34)
Half siblings			
Headache	5.3	11.7	5.9
Neck	5.8	11.2	5.5
Back	6.6	12.6	6.0
Muscle	5.8	10.9	4.8
Chest	6.9	11.7	5.4
Joint	5.5	10.6	6.0
Total	36.2	69.3	38.9
	Father (n = 32)	Mother (n = 32)	Sibling (n = 32)
Step siblings			
Headache	6.4	11.4	6.9
Neck	6.9	12.1	6.8
Back	7.6	12.7	7.4
Muscle	6.3	11.3	6.7
Chest	6.7	10.4	6.4
Joint	6.6	10.9	6.5
Total	40.5	68.1	40.8

[a]Scores range from −42 top 156.

PARENTING STYLES WITH HIGH CORPORAL PUNISHMENT AS A FACTOR IN PAIN REPORTS IN YOUNG ADULTS

The proposition that somatic pain in young adults can be an expression of childhood neglect and abuse has been proposed by Engel (1959). Violon (1985) and Violon and Giurgea (1983) suggest that nonorganic pain in adults is frequently related to childhood abuse and neglect. However, the fact remains that psychological abuse does not invariably lead to somatizing behavior. The pain literature has not previously assessed the impact of punitive parental practices of discipline and current pain reporting. The results of Berger, Knutson, Mehm, and Perkins (1988) showed that their sample, which consisted primarily of middle-class young adults, had experienced a wide range of physical discipline during childhood. Over 12% of their sample described being injured by the discipline of their parents and identified the specific injuries. It is interesting to note that even though 12.1% of respondents identified themselves as being injured by parents, fewer than 3% of respondents labeled themselves as having been physically abused as a child. This suggests a disparity between what one considers to have been abuse toward oneself and professional or public criteria for abuse. Of those who received broken bones, only 43% classified themselves as being physically abused. Also, only 35–38% of those receiving burns, cuts, dental injuries, or head injuries classified themselves as physically abused.

Marykuca (1994) investigated the relationship between abuse and pain in a young, nonclinical population ($N = 409$) of first-year university students. He reported that the perception of having had a punitive childhood was not significantly related to current pain reports in a young adult university student population.

In a collateral study by Roy, Marykuca, Thomas, and Cook (1993), the association between childhood abuse and complaints of pain was investigated. A survey of 409 first-year university students yielded 18 abused persons. They were closely matched for demographic characteristics with 18 nonabused students. The two groups were compared for presence of pain problems, their severity, and methods of treatment. The 18 abused subjects were 4.4% of the total sample. This figure is higher than prevalence of self-rated abuse in the student population in the normative group for surveys. Pain as an ongoing symptom was relatively common in both groups. The following pain sites were reported by the abused and the nonabused students, respectively: back pain, 33% and 44%; headache, 44% and 28%; neck, 22% and 17%; muscle, 22% and 28%; joint, 28% and 39%; stomach, 17% and 11%; and internal pain, 11% and 6%. The average duration of pain for the abused group was 57 months, with a range of 3 to 192 months. For the control group, the mean duration of pain was 46 months, with a range of 4 to 99 months. These differences were nonsignificant, although the trend was for the abused group to report longer duration of pain. Overall, in a young adult nonclinical but abused group, reported pain was not more prevalent than in a matched control group. In this instance it would appear that negative life events do not necessarily have an impact through modifying pain behaviors.

MEMORY AS A FACTOR INFLUENCING PREVALENCE OF PAIN REPORTS IN YOUNG ADULTS

One mechanism that links life events, transition periods, and current pain functioning in young adults is their memory for childhood and adolescence. Retrospective reports of pain are almost universal as the method of data collection for prevalence rates of pain in epidemiological studies with all age groups and not just young adults. However, reliability of memory becomes a critical methodological issue as time increases between earlier life events and the recall of that event. Life transitions are an ongoing process that do not interact uniformly across individuals.

Research has found that typically an adult's earliest memories are reported as being from between the third and fourth years of childhood (Kihlstrom & Harackiewicz, 1982). Memories are usually incomplete before the age of 7, and those that are remembered are often linked to some event that is of personal significance.

Heuer and Reisberg (1990) have suggested that memory for painful events is susceptible to change. Clearly, the turbulence of life transitions would be a factor capable of metamorphosing memories of previous pain experiences. Kihlstrom and Harackiewicz (1982) found that one characteristic of unpleasant and traumatic memories is that they are quite susceptible to change. In contrast, Conway (1990) reported that vivid memories, which include pain memories, seem to be consistent over time. Christianson and Loftus (1990) looked at the characteristics of traumatic memory in which painful physical events were considered. They found that individuals exhibited relatively accurate memory for the central details of an emotional event but inaccurate recollection of the details surrounding the event.

One study on memory for everyday painful events compared young adult university students and seniors from the general community for worst pain memories (Roy, Thomas, & Makarenko, 1990). It was found that both groups had a tendency to recall more recent pain events as more painful than past pain events. It was also found that when a pain memory was recalled from the past, it was usually associated with something traumatic, emotional, or meaningful. These findings are consistent with those reported by Usher and Neisser (1993) that being hospitalized during the third and fourth years of life persisted into adult memory. Morley (1993) found that of memories for everyday events, vivid memories of painful events were the most easily retrieved.

Studies suggest that postevent information can be a factor that leads to the inability to accurately remember an original event (Belli, 1989; Loftus & Hoffman, 1989; Weinberg, Wadsworth, & Baron, 1983). The literature also suggests credibility of the individual presenting misleading information is another important factor that must be considered when examining the influence of suggestion on memory (McGinnies & Ward, 1980).

Thomas et al., in an unpublished work presented at the Canadian Psychological Association Annual Conference in 1996, reported on the influence of suggestion of pain location and the credibility of the suggestion source on memory for the most physically painful event before the age of 10. Young adult university students received a suggestion from a high- or low-credible source of either a neutral, head, or stomach location as the most common location for childhood pain. Subjects then reported their memory for their worst pain before age 10.

The sample consisted of 111 students (49 males and 62 females) ranging in age from 18 to 39 years. In addition, a random subsample of mothers (25%) were given questionnaires to verify the participant's reports of past traumatic pain in childhood. Findings indicated a significant inverse correlation between memory and suggestibility. However, memory and suggestibility were not significantly correlated with suggested pain location. In 25% of the subjects, responses were compared to mothers' responses; 70% of the mothers indicated the same location for worst pain before age 10 of pain as the young adults reported from their memory.

The results from the study did not support the hypothesis that prevalence rates of retrospectively reported pain in young adults were significantly influenced by postevent factors such as suggestion. The inverse relationship between memory and suggestibility suggested that if reported pain prevalence rates are unreliable, then it most likely occurs with subjects with poor memories who tended to be more susceptible to suggestion than those subjects with good memories.

CONCLUSIONS

Pain is a multidimensional concept with physical, biochemical, neurological and psychological aspects, as well as context influences such as life events and transition factors. Because the phenomenon of pain is complex, the theoretical understanding of the physical mechanisms underlying pain often differ from patients' perceptions of the experience (Benjamin et al., 1988). Given this complexity, there are a number of contextual factors such as family stability and form, childhood discipline practices, and memory for past pain experiences that appear capable of influencing the reported prevalence rates at different locations for pain in young adults. Only recently have studies investigating distribution of reported pain in young adults included general populations rather than relying solely on selected clinical samples (Jack, 1981; Sternbach, 1986a,b).

The demographics of the young adult samples investigated in the series of studies reported by Thomas (1993a) do not lend themselves to direct comparisons with most chronic pain populations. With this caution, the young adult multisamples of university students and their siblings still reported high frequencies of weekly pain. The high levels of pain reported were of particular interest: current pain, 25%, while pain during the past week exceeded 60%. The report of one of four university students experiencing pain at some location at any given time indicates this age group has frequent pain, which is consistent with the average in previous studies, which ranged from 15% (Sternbach, 1986a) to 20% (Roy, Thomas, & Makarenko, 1990).

The psychological and disability scores for these students, however, suggest that the pain experienced is minimally disruptive to their daily functioning. These findings suggest that frequent and/or "chronic" pain experiences are more common than thought in young adults, but that high pain frequency is not necessarily associated with psychological pathology or daily functional disability. For all samples reported by Thomas (1993a), headache, muscle, and back pain were the most frequent locations of reported pain and chest pain was the least frequently reported pain location. Thus, the reported pain frequencies by location in this study continue to contradict the view that normative health in a general sample of young adults is generally pain free.

In conclusion, the sibling subjects in this study appear to be a representative nonclinical pain sample of this age group in their reported pain frequencies and locations. However, interpretation of the findings from these series of studies is limited in its generalizability because the samples were drawn primarily from a university population. Also, the data from all the siblings in the families were not assessed; only data from those siblings closest in age to the university part of the sample were assessed (the average number of siblings in the families surveyed was slightly greater than three). Thus, the representativeness of the data from the reporting sibling pairs in a family is unknown. Even with the limitations in this study, the findings still strongly suggest that pain reports are not randomly distributed in sibling pairs of young adults in a nonclinical population.

The results in this study also appeared nonsupportive of a direct genetic explanation as a general theoretical family factor that explains the highly similar pain patterns found in the siblings. The findings further seem to indicate that family sympathy is not significantly related to pain locations most frequently reported by young adults in this sample. However, there were a number of findings that were consistent with the theoretical view that past life events and current life transition processes likely have a role (as yet most undefined by direct research findings) in pain behaviors in young adults.

Although attendance is greatest at pain clinics during middle age, the origin of the ongoing patterns of pain complaints would appear to be during adolescence and young adulthood (Thomas, 1994; Thomas & Roy, 1995). Without longitudinal studies, there is no certainty that those individuals who report frequent pains during adolescence and young adulthood will eventually be the group from whom individuals who will develop chronic pain. At this time it is evident that pain complaints are focused within families rather than randomly distributed individually. This finding, however, still allows understanding of the relative importance of various categories of variables such as genetic–biological vulnerability and social learning such as family modeling or reinforcement versus individual dispositions such as depression and/or somatic anxieties for young adults. The findings in this chapter do suggest, however, that etiologic understanding of chronic pain in middle age will likely need to take a longer time–age perspective and to see chronic pain as a pattern that is likely present far earlier than previously thought. The mechanisms of how the earlier subclinical patterns of pain and accompanying psychological dysfunction transform into chronic pain, however, is still to be determined.

CHAPTER 4

Chronic Pain and Family Functioning in College Students

Entering university is an enormous transition in the lives of most young people. The extent of change is determined by a number of factors such as leaving home or even going to another country and culture. University life itself is quite different from high school and demands a great deal of adaptive skills to adjust to an environment where the student has an unprecedented level of personal freedom. A quick search reveals a burgeoning literature on family-related stress issues for college students. These issues cover a wide spectrum, ranging from withdrawing from university (Sartoris & Vanderwell, 1981) to parental financial support (Bunnett, 1975) to psychological problems in students (Teoh, 1974). Health problems for students related to life events have also come under scrutiny (Anderson & Arnoult, 1989; Bunce, Larsen, & Peterson, 1995; Cohen, Simons, Rose, & McGowan, 1986; Diedricks, 1995; Duckitt & Broll, 1982; Evans, Pitts, & Smith, 1988; Flett, Blankstein, Kirk, Hicken, & Watson, 1995). A few of these studies are briefly discussed.

In a retrospective study of 159 college students, Anderson and Arnoult (1989) found that negative stress (caused by undesirable life events) was directly related to both psychological and physical health as a main effect, but positive stress (caused by desirable events) was not.

The role of social support as a moderator or buffer against negative stress was tested in a population of 77 undergraduates during transition from high school to college (Diedricks, 1995). Negative events were not related to distress symptoms, and the relationship between life events, social support, and psychological symptoms was not clear. An earlier study by Duckitt and Broll (1982), involving 139 students who participated in a prospective study, also failed to confirm the hypothesis that social support had a moderating effect on health impairments due to negative life events.

A prospective study of 30 undergraduate students explored the role of minor life events and onset of minor infections (Evans, Pitts, & Smith, 1988). Students kept a daily journal of desirable and undesirable events, as well as information regarding their physical health. Results showed that compared to carefully matched controlled days, illness episodes were followed by a significant decrease in desirable events of the previous 4 days. This is a rather unique and important study for demonstrating the very short-term effects of lack of positive events and not just the presence of negative events on minor illnesses.

This brief excursion into life events and social support literature points up some existing uncertainties about the protective power of social support to mitigate or obliterate the negative consequences of undesirable life events. On the other hand, some level of consensus on the question of the effects of undesirable life events on health does exist. Yet, a vast majority of students seem to go through this phase without much trial and tribulation. For a few, university life becomes a daily test of will and power of perseverance. Anxiety, especially in the early days of university life, is relatively common.

Over the past 10 years or so, we have conducted a series of studies to investigate many of the social and clinical dimensions of chronic pain in a nonclinical population of university students. In the previous chapter, we discussed some of our more salient findings about the nature and extent of pain. This chapter explores the psychosocial aspects, mainly focusing on the family issues, as they impinge on the overall functioning of the students. It must be stated at the outset that in exploring the pain-related issues in this population we are examining mainly a basically healthy population, who have demonstrated sufficient intellectual and other skills to avail themselves of university education.

Before embarking on the main purpose of this chapter, which is to present and discuss our own research, the broad literature pertaining to the pain and family issues in this population is presented. Surprisingly, the family aspects of college students have not been a popular topic for researchers. The existing literature, albeit slender in scope, examines the family problems of college students from varied perspectives, ranging from general emotional problems to drug addiction to reasons for withdrawal from university education. This literature is presented in the hope that it will acquaint the reader with a general appreciation of family problems encountered by college and university students. The literature review that follows is more of an annotation than a critical review, although serious methodological problems, when called for, will be discussed.

LITERATURE REVIEW

The literature is so disparate that it defies convenient classification. In broad terms, however, it is the population under study that unites them. A few studies have addressed family issues in relation to addiction and health problems in students (Blotcky, 1981; Buelow, 1995; Buelow & Buelow, 1995; Hill, Nord, & Blow, 1992; Siksna, 1988; Wampler, Fischer, Thomas, & Lyness, 1993; Wright & Moore, 1982). These studies tend to confirm that family issues appear to play some role in the drug and alcohol addiction among college students.

Wright and Moore (1982) surveyed 619 undergraduate students. Just over 13% of male and 4.2% of female students reported addiction problems. It should be noted that no independent verification was sought for the students' perceived drug abuse. Both groups showed significant family problems, ranging from parental abuse to parental anger and rejection. For male students, in addition to abuse, drug addiction was significantly related to perceived maternal emotional problems, parental rejection and anger, feelings of boredom, and lack of appreciation by parents. For female students, factors were similar except for maternal drinking. Major methodological flaws in this study were the sole reliance on the survey data and the complete absence of standardized instruments, such as a family functioning scale, to assess with some degree of authenticity and veracity students' self-reports.

A Swedish study involving 190 university students also reported serious family and addiction problems in 36 students, who did not have the necessary qualifications for university entrance but were nonetheless admitted (Siksna, 1988). Compared to other students, this group demonstrated a much higher rate of consultation with the university psychiatric services.

Hill, Nord, and Blow (1992), in a study of alcoholism among 40 adults aged 18 to 30 years (somewhat older age group than university students), assessed the consequences of family history and environment on their drinking. Twenty parents were alcohol dependent and another 20 were social drinkers. Family information was based on an home environment interview.

Parental alcoholism was also investigated by Wampler and colleagues (1993), who examined relationships among addiction in family members, family functioning, which was assessed by Family Adaptability and Cohesion Scale II, and risk estimation for 169 college students. Both family functioning and presence of an alcoholic parent contributed significantly to offspring alcoholism. However, alcoholism in a parent showed a direct relationship with a high risk of alcoholism in their children. Family functioning was an indirect risk. High levels of drinking were noted in both parents and childen. Yet, the most significant family factor related to alcohol abuse was parental alcoholism. Abusive punishment and poor emotional health also emerged as significant factors with the alcohol-dependent students. The authors concluded that the environmental interactions with alcohol-dependent parents were the most powerful predictors of alcohol abuse in young people.

Two studies were conducted by Buelow (1995) and Buelow and Buelow (1995). Buelow and Buelow (1995) examined the gender differences in the etiology and consequences of drug abuse in 28 female and 25 male undergraduates. The Family Function Inventory was used to assess family-related problems. No significant differences emerged between the two groups. As for the consequences, male subjects were more likely to neglect their duties, whereas women ran the risk of blacking out and losing friends.

In the second study, Buelow (1995) investigated family relations, college adjustment, and chemical dependence in 245 college students. These students were divided into three groups: (1) homes with serious drug dependency problem, (2) dysfunctional homes where addiction was not an issue, and (3) nonabusive and well-functioning families. Among other measures, the Family Function Inventory and the Role Relationship Inventory were used. Slowed adult role assimilation in families emerged as a significant predictor for alcohol and drug abuse. Children were also more likely to encounter problems in their transition to adult roles.

Finally, in a study of 72 university students, Blotcky (1981) found that family dysfunction was a major contributory factor in the duration of physical health problems, but was not significant in the etiology of physical illness. This study was correlational, and while showing an interesting association between family dysfunction and ill health, the mechanisms involved in that process were not self-evident.

The family literature on the university student population is limited. In this overview, we have tried to show that family dysfunction due to health and social problems is not uncommon. In the remainder of this chapter, we shall present our research, spanning some 10 years, on pain and family issues in an university (nonclinical) population. As was evident from the previous chapter, our work with this population involves several samples, although all were drawn from first-year university students. For that reason, we shall present six previously published studies, and each will be discussed in some detail. In the final section of this chapter, we shall synthesize our major findings.

THE STUDIES

Study 1

In our first study in this series, we surveyed 18 freshman from an introductory psychology course (Roy, Thomas, & Cook, 1991). These students were selected from a larger population of students and both parents who were headache sufferers. This study population consisted of 18 mothers, 18 fathers, and 18 first-year university students. Twelve of the students were female and six male. The mean age of the mothers was 35.7 and fathers 44.5. The mean age of the students was 20 years. The average family income was $49,510.00 per annum (SD = 28.76). The purpose of the study was to investigate the impact of headache when more than one member of the family suffered from headache.

Measures. Measures used across most of the studies discussed below were the same with some variations. (1) A demographic and health questionnaire (developed by ourselves) was used. (2) The Family Assessment Measure (FAM), which consists of 50 items and has nine subscales was used. The subscales are task accomplishment, role performance, role performance, communication, affective expression, affective involvement, control, values and norms, social desirability, and denial (Skinner, Steinhauer, & Santa-Barbara, 1983). FAM was developed using a large sample of normal and clinical families and has the capacity to differentiate significantly between clinical and nonclinical families. (3) The Visual Analog Scale (VAS) has been used extensively to measure pain intensity in clinical research and has been shown to have high degree of reliability and validity (Huskisson, 1983). Finally, (4) the Beck Depression Inventory, Standard Form (BDI), which consists of 17 sets of statements was used. Answers are provided on a Likert-type scale for each section, ranging from absence of the problem to extreme problem (Beck & Beamesdefer, 1974). The BDI is probably the most common instrument used to measure depression in the pain literature.

Results. Respondents were asked to report the number of headaches they had during the previous 4 weeks. Mothers reported 3.4 episodes (SD = 1.17), fathers 2.5 (SD = 1.21), and students 4.4 (SD = 5.13). On the VAS, the headache emerged to be of a mild nature. Mothers reported a pain intensity of 2.75 (SD = 2.8), fathers 2.0 (SD = 2.28), and students 1.8 (SD = 1.72). Despite these low levels of pain, use of medication was reported by 23.5% of mothers, 22.5% of fathers, and 27.5% of the students. Alcohol to control pain was used by 11.8% of fathers, 18.8% of the students, and none by mothers. On the BDI, all but one of the population scored well below the clinical range of 21.

On the FAM, scores between 30 and 40 suggests family strength, between 40 and 60, average family functioning and score 60 represents family problems. The families in this study presented a very complex picture:

1. In relation to Task Accomplishment, which determines the families' capability to meet certain tasks, the participants scored near the 50 mark, thus suggesting average family functioning in this area. Role Performance assesses two tasks: (1) assignment of specific tasks, and (2) the actual execution of the tasks. On this scale, all three groups scored on the borderline of 60, on the border of "average" and "problem" functioning.
2. As for Communication, which is the only means of exchanging information, all three groups scored from the low to the high end of 60s, thus revealing difficulties with Communication. In Affective Expression, which addresses the feeling component of family life, students were functioning on the borderline of average and problem range, but both groups of parents scored over 60, thus placing their Affective Expression in the problem category.
3. The task of Involvement determines the quality of involvement family members have with each other, which can help or hinder the accomplishment of tasks. This was a very problematic area for all subjects, as all of them scored around 65, the "problem" range of FAM.
4. Control is defined as the process by which family members influence one another. This aspect shows the predictability and consistency of family life as well as the constructive feelings of responsibility for one another. Control emerged as a highly problematic area for these 18 families, with scores in the high 60s.
5. The Values and Norms, which examines family rules, flexibility with which these rules are implemented, and, importantly, consistency of family norms with cultural norms. All three groups scored in the high 60s, revealing an elevated level of disaffection and difficulties in this very critical area.
6. Social Desirability and Denial scores tend to be higher for non-problem families. On both dimensions, the families scored in the low 50s, demonstrating an average level of problems (Table 4.1).

It must be recognized that this was a very preliminary study, without the benefit of a control group. The findings, however, re-

Table 4.1. FAM Score of Student and Parents

FAM scales	Students	Mothers	Fathers
Task Accomplishment	49.67 (SD = 5.4)	49.11 (SD = 3.6)	50.22 (SD = 6.9)
Role Performance	60.61 (SD = 6.4)	59.22 (SD = 4.7)	58.11 (SD = 6.9)
Communication	63.94 (SD = 10.25)	67.28 (SD = 7.00)	64.67 (SD = 8.8)
Affective Expression	59.39 (SD = 5.5)	61.67 (SD = 7.1)	61.00 (SD = 7.8)
Involvement	65.67 (SD = 4.3)	65.44 (SD = 4.7)	65.72 (SD = 3.7)
Control	69.67 (SD = 7.5)	68.89 (SD = 7.9)	69.11 (SD = 5.00)
Values and Norms	68.56 (SD = 10.9)	68.72 (SD = 7.1)	68.94 (SD = 8.3)
Social Desirability	52.61 (SD = 4.9)	54.39 (SD = 3.5)	53.00 (SD = 4.8)
Denial	56.89 (SD = 7.3)	59.39 (SD = 6.1)	58.94 (SD = 6.00)

vealed a number of interesting facts. The most critical finding was that while pain problem itself was of a nominal kind, family problems encountered by these 18 families bordered on serious. It may be surmised that the late adolescence phase of the students combined with the advent of middle age, especially in the fathers, created a period of strain in the families. This study failed to establish any direct relationship between headache and overall family functioning, other than to note that late adolescence, middle-age parents, and headache in all three may contribute to an unhappy home.

Study 2

In this study, we broadened the scope of our investigation, first by increasing the number of subjects and adding a measure to assess illness behavior (Thomas, Roy, & Cook, 1991). Our sample comprised 145 college students and 55 of their parents. As we reported in the previous study, the parent sample was composed of both parents of 18 students; for this study, an additional 19 students, whose one parent agreed to take part in this study, were added. Parents of the remaining 108 subjects declined our invitation. All students and participating parents completed the standard health and demographic questionnaire and the following questionnaires: the BDI, FAM, and VAS.

The demographic profile for this group was similar to the previous group. As for pain, we investigated presence of headaches as well as back pain during the previous 4 weeks. The parent group (N = 55) reported having 2.78 episodes of backache (SD = 3.31) and 2.82 headaches (SD = 1.46). During the same period students recorded 3.07 episodes of backache (SD = 5.82) and 3.7 episodes of headaches (SD = 2.7). These differences failed to attain statistical significance.

Nearly 70% of the parents and 62% of the students knew the diagnosis of their pain-related conditions. At least one quarter of both groups had received treatment for pain and 26.3% of parents and 17.04% of students were on analgesic medications. Alcohol use to control pain was reported by 7.3% parents and 12.76% students. Statistically significant differences were found on all of the above factors. On the VAS, both groups reported very mild pain. Parents and students scored well below the clinical range on the BDI.

The final area of investigation was family functioning. We shall report our findings in two different ways. First, overall comparison of all students and all parents, and second, 19 students where one parent responded. We have already presented our findings on the 18 students and their parents.

In the following areas the parents and the students were functioning in the average range of the FAM: Task Accomplishment, Role Performance, Affective Expression, Social Desirability, and Denial. On the Communication scale, both groups scored in the "family problem" range. Involvement, Control, and Values and Norms were all in the problem range for both groups.

It is noteworthy that compared to the FAM profile of 18 students and their parents, the profile of this group was not dissimilar, except that the former's profile indicated higher levels of problems. The FAM profile for 19 students and 19 parents was remarkably similar to the others. Communication, Involvement, and Control were all in the "family problem" range (Table 4.2).

The FAM score of 145 students is worthy of attention (Table 4.2). In keeping with the general pattern, family functioning in the areas of Communication, Involvement, and Value and Norms were in the problem range. These scores were compatible with the overall pattern of all groups (Table 4.2). This observation strengthens the argument that family problems may be endemic in this age group with or without pain. The task ahead is to explore in more specific terms the impact if any of pain on family functioning.

Table 4.2. FAM Factor Medians and Standard Deviations

FAM scales	Parents (n = 55)	Students (n = 145)	Parents (n = 19)	Students (n = 19)	M(18)	F(18)	S(18)
Task accomplishment	49.2	49.89	48.27	50.63	49.11	50.22	49.67
	SD 5.18	5.34	4.99	4.52	3.6	6.97	5.5
Role performance	57.36	58.17	54.77	56.10	59.22	58.11	60.61
	6.35	7.25	8.14	8.03	4.7	6.1	6.4
Communication	64.32	66.43	61.05	69.57	67.28	64.67	63.54
	8.01	7.94	8.09	5.49	7.00	8.8	10.25
Affective expression	60.47	57.31	58.77	57.63	61.67	61.00	59.29
	6.9	6.85	5.71	7.85	7.1	7.8	5.5
Involvement	65.22	65.51	65.50	64.42	65.44	65.72	65.67
	4.28	4.99	4.28	4.58	4.7	3.7	4.3
Control	67.99	67.95	66.0	67.36	68.89	69.11	69.67
	6.20	7.43	5.68	6.75	7.9	5.00	7.5
Values and norms	68.25	63.35	67.11	71.32	68.72	68.94	68.56
	8.42	9.93	9.73	9.51	7.1	8.3	10.9
Social desirability	53.31	52.49	52.55	53.00	54.39	53.00	52.1
	4.52	5.09	5.15	5.08	3.5	4.8	4.5
Denial	58.51	56.84	57.22	55.52	59.39	58.94	56.89
	6.69	8.22	7.87	9.93	6.1	6.00	7.3

Study 3

In the final study in this group, we compared university students and their siblings with and without headache (Roy, Thomas, & Cook, 1996). The purpose again was to investigate whether the presence of pain in the students and one of their siblings impacted family functioning. A matched control group was established for comparison.

Subjects were 34 pairs of biological siblings, both reporting headaches during the previous week, and a comparison group of 16 pairs of biological siblings who did not report any headaches during the previous week. All subjects completed the demographic questionnaire as well as the FAM and the Family Environment Scale (FES). FES is a well-tested instrument that measures family function, but the properties are somewhat different from FAM. *T* tests and discriminate function analyses were used for data analyses.

The findings of the study corroborated results from the two earlier studies, showing that pain tends to be of low intensity. Family functioning in the headache and nonheadache groups on the FAM was less problematic than the previous two studies. On only one scale—Affective Involvement—the siblings in the nonheadache group scored in the family problem range (Table 4.3). However, the differences between the two groups of FAM failed to attain statistically significant values. Scores were also very similar between the two groups on FES (Table 4.4).

The most intriguing aspects of this study was that discriminant function analyses based on 20 scores of family functioning (10 from FAM and 10 from FES) revealed that siblings from headache families could be predicted with 97.33% accuracy. Again, using the same test based on 20 scores of family functioning, it was found that siblings from nonheadache families could be predicted with 92.59% accuracy.

In the first two of these studies, several points are worthy of attention. First and foremost, these preliminary studies were conducted with the objective of exploring the relationship between pain in a nonclinical population and its effect(s), if any, on family functioning. On measures of pain and psychopathology, students and their parents emerged as relatively healthy. They suffered from mild pain, and depression was conspicuous by its absence. Yet, the family profiles revealed a pattern of common areas of problems. It is quite

Table 4.3. Family Functioning Scores

Family Assessment Measure (FAM)[a]	Means of siblings with headaches	Means of siblings without headaches
Task accomplishment	6.64	6.30
	56.20	54.50
Role performance	6.70	7.04
	54.50	56.20
Communication	6.46	7.00
	56.30	59.00
Affective expression	6.67	7.59
	56.68	60.95
Affective involvement	4.98	6.74
	53.92	61.96
Control	5.95	4.81
	55.75	50.05*
Values and norms	6.46	6.04
	57.84	56.16
Social desirability	8.89	9.44
	46.67	47.88
Defensiveness	7.90	8.74
	41.70	44.96
Total	59.59	53.00*

[a]No significant difference emerged between the two groups in any of the subscales of the Family Assessment Measure.
$^{*}P > 0.06$.

Table 4.4. Family Functioning Scores

Family Environment Scale (FES)	Means of siblings with headaches	Means of siblings without headaches
Cohesion	7.21	9.89
Expressiveness	5.08	7.30
Conflict	3.95	5.41
Achievement orientation	5.75	6.04
Intellectual–cultural orientation	5.45	4.89
Independence	6.50	6.32
Moral religious emphasis	4.77	4.96
Active recreational	6.24	5.21[a]
Organization	4.98	5.93[a]
Control	4.65	4.82

[a]$P > 0.05$.

feasible that family problems revealed by these studies are not atypical in this population in general. The other possibility is that even mild pain in several members of the family is capable of engendering family conflicts.

The patterns of family functioning revealed by these studies led us to the tentative conclusion that, perhaps in spite of pain complaints and not because of them, family issues encountered by young adults attending university were problematic. Perhaps life transition problems were major contributory factors to family dysfunction.

Study 3 did have a control group, but the study population was different. Students and their siblings, unlike their parents in studies 1 and 2, were the subjects. Yet, their family functioning both on FAM and FES were in the average and functional ranges of those scales. On the other hand, family functioning was found to be a powerful discriminating factor in predicting families with members with frequent headaches from families with infrequent headaches. Explanation for this is not self-evident. Perhaps those families where pain is a family affair, at least when siblings are involved, learn to adapt and cope with it in a more effective manner. This proposition is tentative at best as we found no evidence of effective family coping in studies 1 and 2, where pain was very much a family affair. Nevertheless, the most important finding of this particular study was the predictive power of family functioning with frequent sibling headaches from those without. From that perspective, the value of investigating family functioning is reiterated.

In the following section, we wish to report three studies from rather varied perspectives involving students and their family members. These studies encompass issues beyond family functioning. For that reason, we shall focus, to the extent possible, only on family-related issues.

Study 4

In the first of these studies we investigated the expression of pain behaviors in young adults from a learning perspective (Thomas, Roy, & Cook, 1992). The influence of family models on pain in one or both parents was explored. Subjects were 141 first-year university students. For 33 students (23%), a family subsample of parents (33 pairs of mothers and fathers) provided a validity check for students' perception of family members' pain frequency and severity.

All students were administered an expanded questionnaire modified from one developed by Prohaska, Laventhal, Laventhal, and Keller (1985). One or more parents of 67 students (47.5%) returned completed questionnaires. Both parents of 33 students also responded. Respondents rated their pain and illness experiences and their perception of each other family member's pain for ten categories: (1) headache, (2) neck pain, (3) back pain, (4) muscle pain, (5) chest pain, (6) stomach pain, (7) joint pain, (8) tooth- or earache, (9) nausea, and (10) cramps. An expanded demographic and health questionnaire included questions of pain attribution regarding family members and personal experiences with pain.

Results. Selected demographic data were compared between the student subjects without cross-validated family data and with a student subsample with cross-validated family data using descriptive statistics (Table 4.5). The proportion of males and females between the sample and smaller subsample was the only significantly different variable. About 50% of the subjects reported current pain (past 24 h), the most common of which was headache. Surprisingly, 18% students reported chronic pain of 1 to 5 years' duration.

The students reported that on average one (mean = 0.98) family member was concurrently experiencing pain. Of those with concurrent pain, 39.4% were mothers, 18.3% fathers, and rest were siblings. Intensity of pain was of a mild nature for all groups.

A descriptive analyses of the parental subsample determined that the mean age of the parents was 47 years. The fathers were on

Table 4.5. Ratings of Students' Perceptions of Family Expression of Pain[a]

	Fathers Mean/SD	Students Mean/SD	Mothers Mean/SD
Likelihood of visits to doctors for pain	18.16/06.5	19.94/08.2	16.86/07.5
Likelihood of missing work due to pain	18.41/07.1	17.45/08.8	15.88/07.5
Likelihood of taking medication for pain	22.27/08.3	25.40/09.9	21.58/10.0

[a]Scores range from 10 to 50 (sum of 10 pain categories).

average slightly more than 4 years older than the mothers. Parents reported less current pain (41.2%) than the students (49.6%). A series of preplanned *t*-tests were conducted to determine if the students perceived major differences for family members in their pain-related behaviors (Table 4.5). Students perceived fathers to be significantly less likely to engage in pain behaviors. Fathers were perceived by students in comparison to mothers as having: (1) significantly ($P <$ 0.01) less pain in a month; (2) significantly ($P < 0.0001$) less likely to visit a doctor for pain; (3) significantly ($P < 0.0001$) less likely to miss work because of pain; (4) significantly ($P < 0.0001$) less likely to take medication for pain; and (5) in general, significantly ($P < 0.01$) less sensitive to pain.

Students perceived only two differences between themselves and their mothers in relation to expression of pain behaviors. Mothers were perceived as significantly ($P < 0.05$) more likely to visit doctors for pain and significantly ($P < 0.005$) more likely to take medication. Finally, students described themselves as significantly ($P < 0.001$) more likely to miss work because of pain than fathers. Students and fathers reported being most influenced in their attitudes and beliefs about pain and illness by personal experiences and family interaction (Table 4.5). In contrast, mothers as a group reported being most influenced about pain and illness by personal experience and interaction with medical professionals.

Finally, a series of multiple regressions were conducted using data derived from 33 students and 66 parents. The dependent variable was an index of self-initiated expressions of pain complaints. The behaviors in the index were: (1) taking medication, (2) missing work or university, and (3) visiting a physician. The results for students was a regression correlation of $R^2 = 0.32$ (df = 2,24, $F = 5.62$, $P <$ 0.01). Only two variables reached significance for predicting student expression of pain behaviors: (1) fathers' expressive pain behaviors (F = 8.10, df = 1,25, $P < 0.01$) and (2) and the students' perception of the severity of their fathers' pain (F = 2.62, df = 2,24, $P < 0.12$) (Table 4.6).

The best regression correlation combination for predicting male students' pain behaviors was $R^2 = 0.70$ (df = 33,7, $P < 0.05$). Three individual variables were significant in predicting students' expressive pain behaviors: (1) students' perception of the severity of their mothers' pain ($F = 5.73$, df = 1,9, $P < 0.05$); (2) fathers' pain behaviors

Table 4.6. Stepwise Multiple Regression Model for Students' Pain Behaviors in Response to Pain[a]

	df	*f*	Significance
Students' perception of fathers' behavior towards pain	1,15	17.40	$P < 0.001$
Students' perception of mothers' behavior towards pain	2,14	5.01	$P < 0.05$
Students' perception of fathers' severity of pain	3,13	2.49	$P < 0.14$
Fathers' own rating of severity of pain	4,12	2.05	$P < 0.18$
Model $R^2 = 0.76$	4,12	9.27	$P < 0.01$

[a]$N = 33$.

($F = 2.02$, df = 2,8, $P < 0.20$); and (3) mothers' self-rating of pain severity ($F = 4.38$, df = 3,7, $P < 0.08$).

The best regression correlation for female students' pain behavior was $R^2 = 0.76$ (df = 4,12, $P < 0.01$). Four individual variables reached significance in correlating with female students' pain behaviors: (1) The female students' perception of their fathers' pain behaviors ($F = 17.40$, df = 1,15, $P < 0.001$); (2) the female students' perception of the mothers' pain behavior ($F = 5.01$, df = 2,14, $P < 0.050$); (3) the female students' perception of their fathers' pain severity ($F = 2.49$, df = 3,13, $P < 0.14$); and (4) the fathers' self-rating of the pain severity ($F = 2.05$, df = 4,12, $P < 0.18$).

It was hypothesized that intergenerational pain modeling would be one of the key mechanisms directly related to reported pain, since the literature has found that chronic pain patients had significantly more pain models in their families. The results from the multiple regressions using the subsample of students and their parents supported the view that students' perception of their parents' pain experiences were as important as the actual presence or absence of pain reported by the parents in predicting the level of pain reported by the student.

Gender of the parent and that of the child emerged as a matter of some importance. The apparent lack of identification by the children with the same-sex parent in the development of similar pain symptoms was an interesting finding. Conceivably, the late adolescence or early adulthood stage of the children could be an important contributory factor in this finding. In a system as complex as a family, the means by which family members influence each other are very complicated. Perhaps, at that stage of development, young adults are more prone to identify with the parent of the opposite gender. Another hypothesis is that an opposite-sex child may elicit greater sympathy and understanding. Our general impression that pain is often a "family" affair in young adults received further confirmation in this study.

Study 5

This study was designed to investigate differences between a typical headache pain group and a no-headache group of young adults using six categories of variables from different perspectives (Thomas & Roy, 1995). The sample consisted of 522 students ranging in age between 17 and 22 years. Self-report of headache intensity and frequency as well as BDI and FAM were used.

Subjects were divided into two equal groups. Analyses consisted of discriminant function analyses and included a univariate comparison of means between the two groups on all the demographic variables. In assessing the family variables, 16 family-related factors (Table 4.7) were able to correctly classify 58% of the subjects in the headache group and 56% of the subjects in the headache-free group. Family function was not significantly different between the two groups.

It is noteworthy that the groups of demographic, psychological, and disability variable were more effective than family functioning, pain behaviors, or childhood health histories in discriminating between university students with headaches from those without. The findings in this study suggest that the order or relative importance of variables in a population of young adult headache subjects may be different than the order of importance for clinical headache populations. For example, the social–biological theoretical perspectives with its focus on the interaction between early developmental phase and learning hypothesizes that childhood pain or illness may indeed predispose individuals to adult pain and disease. This perspective,

Table 4.7. Predicting Headaches Versus No Headache Groups During the Past Week Using Measures of Family Functioning[a]

Variables	R^2	F	Probability $>F$
Family has chronic pain	0.002	1.02	0.3124
Family member being treated for pain	0.001	0.43	0.4300
Father treated for headaches	0.004	2.03	0.1545
Mother treated for headaches	0.006	2.78	0.0961
Brother treated for headaches	0.005	2.53	0.1117
Sister treated for headaches	0.011	5.18	0.0233
FAM			
TA	0.000	0.01	0.9201
RP	0.001	0.79	0.3730
CO	0.000	0.00	0.9677
AE	0.000	0.29	0.5847
AI	0.000	0.15	0.6907
C	0.002	1.12	0.3063
VN	0.001	0.75	0.3860
SD	0.002	1.17	0.2783
D	0.000	0.06	0.8012
FAM Total	0.000	0.00	0.9367

[a]Sixteen variables correctly identified headache 58% ($n = 428$); sixteen variables correctly identified no headaches 56% ($n = 428$).

along with social learning and family function perspectives, was less effective than expected from the clinical literature in discriminating young typical headache sufferers. The implications of these findings, which appear inconsistent with the current emphasis in the clinical research literature, suggest that a similar study using a clinical population would be useful in establishing the relative importance of variables from different perspectives for clinical pain groups as opposed to persistent pain for subjects in each age and sex grouping. Only such studies could determine the extent to which psychological and familial variables might influence head pain in early adulthood.

Study 6

The final study was undertaken to explore the association between childhood abuse and chronic pain in a group of young adults

(Roy et al., 1993). The literature on this association in the clinical chronic pain population is rich, and there is more than tentative evidence for such a relationship (Roy, 1998). We investigated the age of onset of pain and whether such an association indeed commenced before the patients assumed chronic pain status. Our population was nonclinical and consisted of 409 university students with a mean age of just over 20. Of these, 18 subjects reported childhood abuse on the basis of Assessment Environment Questionnaire (Berger et al., 1988). This instrument was developed to investigate experiences of abuse in adolescents and adults. The development of this measure followed the rational statistical approach for producing content validity, with valid items being endorsed and included. The third questionnaire has 164 items that elicit true or false types of responses and is composed of the following 15 scales: Physical Punishment, Father, Mother, Peer Relationships, Perceptions of Discipline, Shared Parenting, Positive Orientation to Education, Age-Appropriate Demands, Marital Discord, Isolation, Community Involvement, Potential Economic Stress, Negative Family Atmosphere, Positive Parental Contact, and Parental Rejection. Subjects endorsing five or more items are considered abused.

Eighteen, or 4.4%, students were identified as abused. These 18 subjects were matched on all key demographic variable with 18 nonabused students. Pain of all kinds was reported by both groups, and on the measure of psychopathology the differences between the two groups were nonsignificant. On FAM, 18 abused–pain subjects functioned in the problem range, whereas the nonabused subjects were in the average range.

Following this initial investigation, which failed to show any particular association between childhood abuse and complaints of pain, we revisited the 18 abused students for a detailed case-by-case analyses (Table 4.8). Two subjects (subjects 1 and 2) reported moderate levels of pain as opposed to the mild pain for the whole group. Both were taking prescription drugs and one was on antidepressant medication. This person, who in all probability had responded well to antidepressant medication, did not score in the clinical range on the BDI. Another subject (subject 3) scored 9 on the VAS, thus recording almost unbearable pain. This subject was resorting to alcohol to control pain. She was also in the clinical range on the Anxiety Scale

Table 4.8. Individual Profiles of Abused Subjects with Pain Problems, Psychological Difficulties, and/or Family Dysfunction

	Subjects				
Variables	1	2	3	4	5
Visual Analog Scale	5	6	9	5	0
Pain duration (months)	0	0	43	3	192
Prescription analgesics	Y	Y	Y	N	Y
Sleep medication	Y	Y	N	N	N
Alcohol for pain	Y	Y	Y	N	N
Antidepressants	Y	N	N	N	N
Anxiety score	14	10	10	9	7
BDI score	1	27	20	12	0
Self-esteem score	25	30	26	27	31
Total disability score	19	—	23	35	7
Total FAM score	62.9	67.6	59.1	67.3	84.7

on the Minnesota Multiphasic Personality Inventory (MMPI). This was the most abused subject in the study on the basis of her score. Subject 4 reported a moderate level of pain on the VAS. There was evidence of disability due to pain in this subject on the basis of the Pain Disability Index. Subject 5, though reporting low pain, had the longest duration of pain (192 months) in the entire sample.

This case-finding approach produced several troubled individuals for whom pain was indeed a serious problem. These findings altered our initial observation that the abused subjects were just as unaffected by pain as the controls. The fact was that at least five (28%) students seemed troubled by a mixture of pain, depression, anxiety, compromised self-esteem, possible alcohol abuse, some disability due to pain, and family dysfunction. Family dysfunction, as measured by the FAM, disclosed that with the exception of role performance, all 18 subjects with history of abuse functioned in the problem range.

Is it possible that childhood abuse could be the genesis of somatic symptoms in later life? Common sense would prompt an affirmative response, and at least the individual profiles of five students showed a tantalizing possibility for the existence of such an association. Our study managed to generate an interesting hypothesis that merits further exploration.

DISCUSSION

We have presented what might appear to be a potpourri of studies. Yet, a common factor linking them together is the family. Family problems in this population of nonclinical pain subjects have not received much attention outside our own studies. Our initial studies indicated moderately serious family difficulties in a population of students with pain problems, albeit of a mild nature, and their parent or parents who also suffered from pain complaints. We were surprised and puzzled by the degree of family dysfunction reported by these families, which seemed incongruent with the degree of pain and the almost total absence of depression. We hypothesized that perhaps the transitional stages of these families combined with "family" pain could be a plausible explanation for the level of family dysfunction. The first two studies were methodologically wanting, as we did not have control groups. In the third study, which did have a control group, the results significantly contradicted the findings related to family functioning of the first two studies. This study investigated pain in the students and their siblings. Family functioning for this group of students and their siblings was on the whole in the average range. The demographic variables for these students were not significantly different than the students in our previous studies.

So, how does one explain the difference? There obviously is no convenient explanation. There was one obvious difference between the subjects of this study and other studies. The latter included students and parents, whereas the former included only siblings. It should be noted, however, that in none of our subsequent studies were we able to replicate the finding related to family function in this particular study. Hence, the differences in the samples may be of some importance. However, for reasons that seem somewhat uncertain, effective family functioning appears to be more of an exception than the rule, at least in the student pain population.

Our disparate group of studies also revealed various levels of family dysfunction. The modeling effect of parental pain was evident in study 4. The gender of the parent emerged as an important factor, as the same-gender (mother–daughter or father–son) modeling effect did not hold in this particular study. Nevertheless, the role of sympathy and identification of children with parents were evident.

Family function or more precisely some aspects of family function emerged as significant in terms of discriminating pain from the nonpain subjects. This study confirmed the power of the learning model as an explanation for pain behavior in young adults. The role of the family in the genesis of pain symptoms received further confirmation.

In the final study, once again upon close scrutiny the role of the family in perpetrating abuse and general family dysfunction revealed the possibility that the abuse–pain relationship has a much earlier beginning than in the middle-aged clinical population. Family factors, for obvious reasons, emerged as of critical importance for understanding and studying this relationship. It is noteworthy that in this study the nonabused group reported family functioning in the average range, which was once again a departure from our previous findings. Whether exclusion of parents from this study influenced the students' perception of family functioning is not clear.

The fact that the family for one reason or another is a critical social system worthy of our attention is neither new nor novel. The proposition lends itself to common sense. From the clinical literature, we are aware of the pervasive negative consequences of chronic pain on the entire family system. In our series of studies, we have merely extended the proposition that the family as an organization is worthy of our attention with a young adult nonclinical pain population. We are left with the impression, supported by some empirical evidence, that even in this relatively healthy group of young adults family factors assume great importance. The nature of the importance remains a matter of some speculation.

PART III

PAIN ISSUES AND MIDDLE AGE

CHAPTER 5

Epidemiology of Chronic Pain and Related Issues in the Middle Years

CHRONIC PAIN AND MIDDLE AGE

There is some recent evidence that when all pain locations are combined that the prevalence of persistent pain reaches its peak (50 to 65%) during middle age (Brattberg et al., 1994; Anderson et al., 1994). These findings would be consistent with data from Von Korff, Dworkin, LeResche, and Kruger (1988), who also found an overall prevalence of 37% of persistent pain in a middle-aged work population. In contrast, several studies have reported that younger adults report more pain than older age groups (Sternbach, 1986a; Thomas & Roy, 1988a), while earlier studies found that the elderly experienced more pain (Crook et al., 1984). Given this inconsistency in the reported epidemiology of chronic or persistent pain, Gibson and Helme (1996) have concluded that at this time the question of which age group is most vulnerable to chronic pain remains moot.

One explanation for the variability in general prevalence rates is changing patterns of vulnerability to chronic pain imbedded within life transition issues across the lifespan. This position is supported by Tibbin et al. (1990), who reported that an interaction between age and pain location and reported prevalences existed; headache and abdominal pain were more frequent locations in younger individuals, a peak for chest and back pain in middle age, and most frequent complaints of joint pain were in the older population.

THEORIES OF PAIN MECHANISMS RELATING TO FIBROMYALGIA

Although important gains in the understanding of the physical mechanisms of pain have been made during the past decade, a gap still remains between physical causes and subjective suffering for many chronic pain patients. In particular, for fibromyalgia the contradiction between the patient's perception of illness and the often rather limited objective findings is stressful (Henriksson, 1995).

Typically, pain syndromes are perceived by the public as having a distinct onset in terms of first appearance of symptoms, life stage when most prevalent, progression of the disorder, etiology, and treatment. This perception in the case of fibromyalgia is significantly inaccurate. Specifically for fibromyalgia, as well as many other types of pain, in a majority of cases the diagnostic workup fails to establish an etiology for the pain (Bonica, 1990; Wall, 1990). According to the International Association for the Study of Pain (IASP) definition, chronic pain is a pain condition that lasts longer than 3 months and is not responsive to treatment. Finally, to further complicate diagnostic classifications, acute recurrent pain, which is similar but not equivalent to either acute or chronic pain, is caused by repeated nociceptive stimulus from a chronic pathological condition such as osteoarthritis (Harkins & Price, 1992).

In the pain literature, various models have been hypothesized to understand pain perception and tolerance. This is especially important in a pain syndrome like fibromyalgia where pain tolerance levels for tenderness to touch is a critical feature for diagnosis. Initial attempts to understand fibromyalgia were mainly from the physiological perspective of muscle inflammation. More recent models have included psychological and experiential aspects in explaining the human experience of pain. The specificity model, or stimulus–response model of pain, states that there are periphery receptors and when they are stimulated as a result of injury to the body, nerve impulses travel through the spinal cord to the brain. The intensity of pain is viewed as a direct reflection of the activity of pain receptors. Various treatment techniques that follow from this theoretical model are more effective for acute type pains but less so for chronic pains (Saxon, 1991). This theoretical pain model offers little explanatory power with regard to possible pain mechanisms for fibromyalgia.

The gate control theory attempts to systematically integrate sensory affective, and cognitive influences on an individual's pain experience. This theory claims that there is a type of gate mechanism in the spinal cord that controls the perception of pain at the spinal cord, subcortical, and cerebral cortical levels. Nociceptors, sensory receptors to pain found in the skin and subcutaneous tissues, are responsive to chemical, thermal, electrical, and mechanical stimulation. These nociceptors are thought to be terminal endings of either A-delta or C nerve fibers. A-delta fibers are larger diameter nerves that relay localized, sharp, pricking pains that are rapidly evoked but of short duration. In contrast, C fibers are small-diameter nerves that relay deep, burning, diffuse dull pains that persist. Finally, A-beta fibers are described as large in diameter and they carry other nonpainful sensory information. All types of nerve fibers send information to the dorsal horn of the spinal cord. From there the stimulus information is transmitted to the thalamus, hypothalamus, limbic system, and cerebral cortex, where the processing actually relating to perception of pain occurs (Harkins, Lagua, Price, & Small, 1995).

The gate mechanism appears to be controlled by the composition of the various types of afferent nerves that have been activated as well as by modulation from the brain and spinal cord. C and A-delta fibers facilitate pain by opening the gate, whereas input from A-beta fibers, resulting from low-threshold mechanoceptors such as touch, appear to suppress the transmission of pain by closing the gate. This theoretical gate can also be influenced to open and close by input from the brain and spinal cord. Thus, this theory allows for emotional and psychological factors to play a part in the perception of pain (Wall, 1990). While the gate theory of pain offers some explanation for specific pain symptoms in fibromyalgia, it provides little predictive power as to which additional symptoms may be concurrent from the diverse possible symptom constellation that is present in fibromyalgia.

Another explanation for the variability in pain perception independent of location and etiology is the presence of neuroregulators in peripheral and central neurons. These chemicals are natural pain moderators that act at the synapses between neurons. Neurotransmitters may be indolamines (i.e., serotonin), catecholamines (i.e., norepinephrine and dopamine), or enkephalins and endorphines. The mechanism of action of these substances is not well understood (Wall,

1990). Studies reporting the use of psychopharmacological agents (cyclic antidepressants, the tricyclic agent cyclobenzaprine, basic molecules, and atypical antidepressants) in the treatment of fibromyalgia show that disturbances in brain neurochemistry are similar for fibromyalgia and major depression. Serotonergic [5-hydroxytryptamine (5-HT)] treatments have been more successful in alleviating pain than depression, whereas catecholaminergic agents have been found to be particularly affective with symptoms associated with depression (Goodnick & Sandoval, 1993). Neurotransmitter changes naturally occur with regularity dependent on age, but typically, marked changes are specific to disease process (for example, dopamine in parkinsonism or acetylcholine in Alzheimer's disease).

Another theoretical explanation of pain mechanisms comes from learning theory. According to this theory there is a distinction between the initial physiological reaction to a painful stimulus and the resulting behaviors. Respondent pain behaviors are conceptualized as actions that result from actual nociception. Operant pain behaviors are actions that develop when the pain experience is linked to forms of reinforcement such as receiving pain medication or attention, or being allowed to avoid unpleasant situations. The association between pain and reinforcement increases the likelihood of the persistence of pain behaviors, which often become separated from the original painful stimulus. If respondent pain behaviors last long enough, learning will occur and behaviors may then be controlled by the operant pain behaviors. In chronic pain both respondent and operant pain behaviors are likely to coexist (Fordyce, 1983; Saxon, 1991).

Since pain is strictly an individual experience, sometimes with limited medical explanations for its frequency, severity, and duration, it is a phenomenon that is almost exclusively dependent on self-reports (Jensen & Karoly, 1992). In self-report studies, individual psychological factors, such as depression (Roy, Thomas, & Matas, 1984; Kerns & Jacob, 1992), and social factors, such as family support (Turk et al., 1987; see also Chapter 6), can interact with biological mechanisms in defining the experience and expression of pain. Social factors such as stoicism and expectations that pain with aging is typical (Cook & Thomas, 1994) provide increasing evidence for an age cohort phenomenon where elderly persons in general report less pain than younger age cohorts (Roy et al., 1990; Thomas & Roy, 1988a). Thus, theoretical explanations for pain must include psychological and social context factors, since pain can be experienced in the absence of organic cause, such as with somatoform disorders. Another psychological factor affecting pain reporting is attention (Bayer, Baer, & Early, 1991). Thus, inclusion of psychological factors as contextual variables surrounding pain increase explanatory power for theories attempting to account for variability in pain reporting across age groups as well as individuals. At the same time, psychological context variables also increase the complexity in understanding pain.

Although pain may begin with a noxious stimulus that can lead to tissue damage, labeling a stimulus as pain still requires interpretation of the physical sensations by an individual. Thus, all self-reported pain experiences must pass through a psychological filter involving cognitive appraisal of the stimulus as well as evaluation of the context in which the stimulus occurs. Additionally, as important as the cognitive component is, the affective dimension of pain is equally critical. Recently, one pain model proposed that the affective dimension of pain is composed of two stages. The first is the immediate emotions related to the actual unpleasant sensations of the pain. The second stage is the evolution of emotional states dependent on subsequent ramifications of experiencing pain that are strongly influenced by subject variables (Price et al., 1992). The longer an individual experiences pain and there is some systematic sign of increased autonomic nervous system activity, the greater the likelihood that the pain experience will be influenced by psychological and social factors. For example, in people with chronic pain due to organic etiology, it is estimated that 20 to 40% experience major depression and another 40% have mood disorders (France & Urban, 1991; Haythornthwaite, Sieber, & Kerns, 1991). Thus, the comorbidity of chronic pain and depression is of continuing research interest. It is currently hypothesized that the relationship is bidirectional. Thus, high levels of depression may result in high levels of reported pain; conversely, high levels of chronicity of pain may lead to development of a major depression (Smith, 1992).

Finally, some researchers specifically postulate that psychological stress triggers physiological pain mechanism involving regional cerebral blood flow (rCBF), cerebral spinal fluid composition (CFS), aberrant auditory brain stem responses (ABR), and oculomotor responses in patients with fibromyalgia (Johansson, Risberg, Rosenhall, Orndahl, et al., 1995). A psychosomatic theory of pain would suggest that specific physical responses are the result of mental stress. Thus, reactions to stress are viewed as involving different neurohormonal aspects that may be both an etiologic factor in the fibromyalgia syndrome and a pathophysiological mechanism that explains the symptoms. This explanation also would be consistent with clinical signs and laboratory findings indicating a central nervous system (CNS) dysfunction in certain cases of fibromyalgia (Johansson, Risberg, Rosenhall, & Orndahl, 1995).

DEFINITION AND HISTORY OF FIBROMYALGIA

The term *fibromyalgia* is descriptive of a condition manifested in widespread musculoskeletal pain that is of chronic duration. The pain must be present in 11 to 18 tender point sites on digital palpation (Caudill, 1995). What differentiates fibromyalgia (FM) from other pain conditions is the widespread configuration of pain locations and the presence of a stage four sleep disruption, resulting in chronic fatigue (Wolfe, Smythe, Yunus, & Bennett, 1990). FM patients frequently experience muscle spasms, headache, poor or nonrestorative sleep, and depressive symptoms. Morning stiffness is often present (Baumstark & Buckelew, 1992). The widespread pain is described as a constant feeling of overexertion and is typically accompanied by a constellation of other diverse symptoms. These include conditions such as irritable bowel syndrome and Raynaud's phenomenon.

The following are the formal diagnostic criteria for fibromyalgia syndrome according to the 1990 Multicenter Criteria Committee (Wolfe et al., 1990):

1. Widespread pain of at least 3 months' duration.
2. Pain in 11 of the following 18 point sites on digital palpation with a pressure of 4 kg.
   a. Occiput: at the suboccipital muscle insertions (bilateral).
   b. Low cervical: at the anterior aspect of the intertransverse spaces at C5–C7 (bilateral).

c. Trapezius: at the midpoint of the upper border (bilateral).
d. Supraspinatus: at origins above the scapula spine near the medial border (bilateral).
e. Second rib: at the second costochondral junctions, just lateral to the junctions on the upper surfaces (bilateral).
f. Lateral epicondyle: 2 cm distal to the epicondyle (bilateral).
g. Gluteal: in upper outer quadrants of buttocks in anterior fold of muscles (bilateral).
h. Greater trochanter: posterior to the trochanteric prominence (bilateral).
i. Knees: at the medial fatpad proximal to the joint line (bilateral).

Because the etiology of FM remains obscure, a definitive course of the illness cannot be predicted. Also, the onset of FM has not been defined. Retrospective reports suggest three forms of onset. The first and most dramatic is onset due to some form of physical trauma. There is limited evidence to suggest that FM resulting from an accident can be and often is more disabling than FM that develops "naturally" (Smiley, Cram, Margoles, Romano, & Stiller, 1992). A second form of onset is related to a protracted physical illness, like influenza. The final and most common type of onset is described as a gradual increase in symptoms over adulthood (Wolfe et al., 1990).

FM was originally conceptualized a *fibrositis*, a term introduced by Gowers in 1904 (Raspe & Croft, 1995). The name, fibrositis, was derived from a constellation of symptoms frequently involving inflammation of fibrous tissues in persons reporting muscle ache (Boissevain & McCain, 1991b). However, muscle biopsies and the response to medical treatments designed to reduce muscle inflammation do not consistently indicate the existence of an inflammatory condition of the muscles in fibromyalgia. Pressure-induced pain sensitivity in FM patients is not most pronounced in muscle tissue and does not depend on increased skin sensibility (Kosek, Ekholm, & Hansson, 1995). Pressure pain and heat pain threshold also have been reported as lower in FM subjects as compared with controls both at tender points and at nontender control points. Also, pain thresholds for electrocutaneous stimuli appear decreased only at tender points and detection thresholds for nonpainful stimuli have been found to be minimally affected in FM. Only tender points have been shown to be more sensitive in individuals with FM than control points for mechanical pressure (Lautenbacher, Rollman, & McCain, 1994).

Many FM symptoms can be categorized as "psychogenic rheumatism." However, the current diagnostic criteria for FM must include the defining pain–sleep relationship in the symptoms and course of the disorder (Smythe & Moldofsky, 1977). Support for the importance of the poor sleep component are shown in a study where FM patients had more alpha electroencephalogram (EEG) sleep and less rapid eye movement (REM) and stage 1 sleep; they were better able to recall their behaviorally signaled awakenings the following morning and reported less satisfying sleep. The heightened vigilant state as indicated by the prominent alpha EEG sleep anomaly probably caused the experience of unrefreshing sleep. Psychological distress demonstrated by more psychopathology than controls in terms of Symptoms Checklist 90 (SCL-90)—Revised scores was also associated with poor sleep (Anch, Lue, MacLean, & Moldofsky, 1991).

It has also been shown that like some forms of depression, FM patients' pain is affected by changes in the weather, including extreme changes in temperature and humidity, stress, anxiety, and poor sleep (Wolfe et al., 1990). As an example of external influences on FM, one recent study (1) examined the relationships among actual weather, disease severity, and symptoms of fibromyalgia; (2) assessed beliefs about weather affecting symptoms; and (3) examined differences between patients with high and low weather sensitivity. Weather affected musculoskeletal symptoms predominantly; however, the strongest relationship was between weather beliefs and self-reported pain such that weather sensitivity tended to be associated with more functional impairment and psychological distress (Hagglund, Deuser, Buckelew, & Hewett et al., 1994).

The challenge associated with the diagnosis of FM is defining it as a medical condition and moving away from the conceptualization that the pain symptoms are purely psychological in origin. Considerable time and effort have been spent differentiating the pain experienced in FM from that described in psychogenic pain conditions. However, current thinking continues to propose a psychobiological relationship between primary FM, major affective disorders, and several other somatoform and psychiatric disorders, possibly suggesting a family of affective spectrum disorders that may be mediated through a common pathway (Tanum & Malt, 1995). FM varies in reported prevalence as a function of the medical specialty of the diagnosing physician, with most frequent diagnosis by rheumatologists, family physicians, and neurologists (Bohr, 1995). From a public perspective, FM as a medical disorder becomes somewhat elusive as individuals suffering from FM may not look "sick," but present a history of pain and disability that is often debilitating.

EPIDEMIOLOGY OF FIBROMYALGIA

Symptoms of FM vary across individuals as well as age groups, with reports of up to 80% of sufferers being women aged 35 to 65 years. FM occurs in roughly 2.1 to 5.7% of the population (Vaeroy, 1996; Wolfe, Ross, Anderson, Russell, & Hebert, 1995), affecting approximately 6% of the North American work force. Characteristic symptomatology includes widespread muscle soreness, fatigue, chronic pain, psychosocial changes, impaired lifestyle functioning, and diminished work capacity (Raymond & Bergland, 1994). Merskey (1996) estimated that FM occurs in women eight to nine times more frequently than in men. Wolfe et al. (1990), in their study of the prevalence and characteristics of FM in a more general population, found rates of FM to be two times higher in the 50–69 age group than in other age groups, although they did identify the presence of FM in all age groups.

COMORBIDITY BETWEEN PSYCHOLOGICAL DISTURBANCE AND FIBROMYALGIA

When reporting the epidemiology of FM, the question of comorbidity of FM and psychological disturbance needs to be addressed in order to better understand the prevalence of the pain syndrome. It has been reported that FM patients tend to minimize or deny psychological symptoms, yet the evidence is overwhelming that comorbidity of psychological disturbances is higher compared with pain complaint controls (Bohr, 1995).

Psychological disturbances were found in 78.5% of women diagnosed with FM (Martinez, Ferraz, Fontana, & Atra, 1995). In the same study, comparisons with randomly selected control patients without chronic muscle pain indicated that personality disturbances were observable in 63,8% of patients and 8% of controls, depression in 80% of the FM patients and 12% of controls, and anxiety in 63.8% of the FM patients and 16% of controls.

Another study evaluated the presence of psychopathology in FM patients compared with control groups of patients with rheumatoid arthritis and patients with lumbar herniation (Krag, Norregaard, Larsen, & Danneskiold-Samsoe, 1994). Patients with FM scored significantly higher than controls on scales of melancholia, atypical depression, and anxiety. Also, the patients with FM scored significantly higher on pain than did controls.

Turning specifically to depression in a study of 327 patients with FM using the Center of Epidemiologic Studies—Depression (CES-D) scale found that employing a cutoff score of 16, which is typically used for the community, 78% of patients were classified as depressed. If a cutoff point of 23 was applied, which according to previous studies indicates clinical depression, the percent of patients affected by depression dropped to 49%; when a cutoff point of 28 was used, 33.8% of patients were diagnosed with severe depression (Ercolani, Trombini, Chattat, Cervini et al., 1994). Likewise, in a study by Ellertsen, Vaeroy, Endresen, Forre (1991), 103 females with FM yielded depression or psychosomatic profile types for 88% of the patients. Other studies have also reported high levels of depression in patients with FM (Krag et al., 1994; Ledingham, Doherty, & Doherty, 1993; Wolfe et al., 1995).

Alfici, Segal, and Landau (1989) even considered that FM was primarily a variant of the depressive disorders. They concluded, however, that while FM patients reported depression on self-rating scales, either in the present or past experiences, their presentation during interviews was not consistently concordant with self-reports. Their results indicated that depressed mood was less apparent in FM patients compared to individuals diagnosed as having major depression. In conclusion, they hypothesized that pain could serve as a substitute for depression, and that somatic preoccupation insulated patients from more severe depression. In a review of the literature, Boissevain and McCain (1991b) also concluded that FM and depression were not a single phenomena representing a unitary dimension. They concluded that while it appears that a significant proportion of FM patients will experience depression in the course of the disorder, depression is not uniformly present and is not unique to FM as a chronic pain condition. This viewpoint would also be consistent with the findings of Buckelew et al. (1994), who reported that 47% of their sample of FM patients met the criteria for possible clinical depression, but that symptoms of depression were not related to pain behaviors.

The primary limiting factor in understanding whether there is a casual relationship between FM and depression and the direction of causality if such a relationship exists is the absence of premorbid data. Without premorbid prevalence rates of depression, one cannot determine the impact of FM on subsequent depression; it has been shown that generally when pain becomes chronic there are reports of depression and when depression becomes problematic reports of pain are more frequent (Reich, Tupin, & Abramowitz, 1983).

DIAGNOSIS AND ASSESSMENT OF FIBROMYALGIA

In attempting to define the etiology of FM, considerable attention has been focused on establishing FM as a distinct medical diagnosis. Comparatively, the differentiation between FM and rheumatoid arthritis is relatively clear and can be determined, given that each has a unique diagnostic constellation of symptoms. Rheumatoid arthritis, a clearly established disease, is characterized by inflammation of the joints and connective tissues. FM is characterized by pain in the muscles of a nonarticular origin. However, because of the similar levels of disability in both conditions, rheumatoid arthritis and FM can have similar psychological symptoms when assessing disability and quality of life (e.g., Martinez, Ferraz, Sato, & Atra, 1995). As with rheumatoid arthritis, diagnostic distinctions between FM and other chronic pain syndromes usually can be made on a physiological basis, although sometimes only with difficulty and after lengthy and careful medical workups. Because of the difficulties encountered in establishing a physical etiology and course of FM, many investigative efforts have focused on determining psychological origins for the disorder.

Clinical studies assessing the psychological characteristics of FM have found strong correlations between FM and somatization scores (Wolfe et al., 1995). Such findings have led some researchers to hypothesize that the pain experienced in FM is a physical manifestation of a psychological disturbance. It is this speculation that has prompted a closer assessment of the symptomatology of FM with respect to the diagnostic criteria for psychological disorders such as hypochondriasis, somatoform pain disorder, and psychogenic rheumatism. Keller (1994) discusses in detail the extent of biological and psychosocial contributions to different psychosomatic syndromes and the relationship of these syndromes to somatization and somatoform disorders. The syndromes in disturbances of physiology summarized included FM, chronic fatigue, motility disorders of the esophagus, nonulcer dyspepsia, irritable bowel syndrome, urethral syndrome, and some defined pain syndromes. It was concluded from the review that the extent of biological and psychosocial contributions vary among these syndromes as well as among individuals with the same syndrome. Many of the phenomena of the somatoform disorders appear to be caused by a clustering of psychosomatic syndromes or their incomplete or atypical manifestations and low sensation thresholds.

Closer examination of the symptom presentation of the psychosomatic syndromes suggests vague and physiologically inconsistent pain complaints that are overly dramatic when described or examined. Many of the pains described tend to mimic other more common pain conditions, like angina (Boissevain & McCain, 1991a). When comparing psychosomatic symptom constellations with those reported by FM patients, Boissevain and McCain (1991b) note that FM symptoms are described and located in a predictable and consistent manner; further, their symptoms are subject to diurnal and weather induced variation. Although FM patients exhibit point tenderness, they may be better able to withstand light pressure than some patients whose pain has a significant psychological component.

Further support for the distinction between FM and psychologically based pain conditions is provided by Dunne and Dunne (1995), who compared FM symptom presentation with diagnostic criteria for somatization disorder and found that generally FM patients would not meet these criteria. In another study (Schoenfeld-Smith, Nicassio, Radojavic & Patterson, 1995), examined whether subgroups of FM patients could be differentiated for one another on the basis of patterns of pain scores, depressive symptoms, and disability. In the study, 118 patients having symptoms for an average of 11.78 years were assessed on these variables and on psychosocial variables hypothesized to influence clinical status, such as social support, helplessness, stress, and coping. A two-cluster solution, identifying a low-functioning group and a high-functioning group, was observed. The low-functioning patients were more impaired in the area of pain, disability, and depression than the high-functioning patients. They tended to be younger and had a lower socioeconomic status than high-functioning patients. The best discriminator of subgroup membership was helplessness.

The relationship between chronic fatigue syndrome and FM also has come under scrutiny. Approximately 75% of FM patients also meet the criteria for chronic fatigue syndrome. Researchers have noted that the two disorders share common features, like headache, muscular weakness, and sleep disturbance (Boissevain & McCain, 1991b). This has led to the proposal that the two disorders share a common etiologic pathway. However, the etiology of chronic fatigue syndrome remains as obscure as FM, so the validity of the assumption remains unsubstantiated (Farrar, Locke, & Kantrowitz, 1995).

In summary, to date there is no generally recognized method of assessing the presence of FM as a medical disorder to the exclusion of other psychosomatic and somatoform syndromes. Not only is there an overlap in reported locations for reported pain and associated other symptoms among a number of somatoform syndromes, but psychological and physiological assessments have not been sufficiently consistent for a definitive diagnosis that specifically guides treatment. Because of the varied symptoms among FM patients in terms of location, pain intensity, psychological impact, and predictable course, there is no uniform agreement as to treatment either medically or psychologically.

NEW DIRECTIONS IN THE TREATMENT OF FIBROMYALGIA

Notwithstanding the absence of clear etiology and course of FM, there is considerable evidence of the impact and disability resulting from the diagnosis. Martinez, Ferraz, Sato, and Atea (1995) concluded that quality of life of FM patients was substantially diminished. Many FM patients have experienced changes in work performance and many are forced to leave full-time employment or to make career changes (MYOPAIN, 1992). Changes in career and employment status often result in downward changes in income levels that are an additional source of stress for patients and families. Not only are income-related duties affected, but many persons with FM are forced to give up hobbies, community activities, and social activities. Furthermore, responsibilities in the home are also affected by the pain of FM. Most FM patients report symptoms that are variable and unpredictable from day to day, resulting in a reluctance to make plans or to look forward to upcoming events (Henriksson, Gundmark, Bengtsson, & Ek, 1992).

The process of living with FM involves taking each day as it comes and focusing on getting through each day without pain exacerbation. Naturally, feelings of self-efficacy are affected by this loss of self-control. Buckelew et al. (1994) noted the presence of a relationship between self-efficacy and pain behavior that they felt emphasized the importance of self-efficacy in successful pain management. Maintaining employment or returning to work for FM patients is particularly difficult. As an example, one study assessed FM patients during the performance of five standardized work tasks, and compared their performance to that of rheumatoid arthritis patients and healthy controls. FM patients performed 58.6% and rheumatoid arthritis patients 62.1% of the work done by controls. Work performance was strongly associated with pretest scores on the disability scale of the Stanford Health Assessment Questionnaire, but also with pain, global severity, and psychological status in both rheumatoid arthritis and FM groups. Work status in 176 FM patients was also examined: 60% were employed; 9.6% considered themselves disabled; but only 6.2% received disability payments (none for the specific diagnosis of FM); and 29% of the FM patients had changed jobs because of their disorder (Cathey, Wolfe, & Kleinheksel, 1988).

The recommended treatment of FM is multimodal and includes relaxation training, biofeedback, physical therapy, and aerobic conditioning. Pharmacological treatment with cyclobenzaprine, amitriptyline, and alprazolam also is recommended (Baumstark & Buckelew, 1992). Also, from a medical perspective the effectiveness and tolerance of *S*-adenosyl-L-methionine (SAMe) in patients with primary FM has been reported positively. SAMe decreased tenderness of painful sites, improved the general sense of well-being, and reduced the mean scores for the Hamilton Rating Scale for Depression, the Self-Rating Depression Scale, the Hamilton Rating Scale for Anxiety, and the Lorish and Maisiak Face Scale (Grassetto & Varotto, 1994).

Another aspect of medical treatment that is receiving more attention in the pain literature with FM is the importance to patients that the treating physician have a supportive attitude toward the psychological stress associated with the disorder. In one study, patients with FM rated their satisfaction with the way each aspect of their treatment had been managed by their physician. Patients whose physician's viewed their psychological concerns as important aspects of treatment were less depressed and/or anxious than patients whose physician's attached less importance to these factors. Patients whose physicians endorsed a broad range of the treatment components tended to experience less sleep disturbance and less disability than did patients whose physician held a less comprehensive view (Potts & Silverman, 1990).

A psychological approach that is being increasingly used due to moderate success in the treatment of pain symptoms in FM patients is hypnosis (Holroyd, 1996). In a recent review, results with FM patients, burn patients undergoing debridement, and cancer patients receiving bone marrow transplants show hypnosis to be an equally or more effective treatment compared to other psychological interventions. Hypnosis is hypothesized to influence the subjective experience of pain. Research suggests that it works through the CNS, peripheral nervous system, or spinal cord down-regulation. It enables modification of cortical responses subsequent to sensory registration and prior to consciousness. Hypnosis effectively reduces chronic pain by lowering anxiety; modifying attitudes, expectations, and beliefs; and improving analgesic suggestibility. In low hypnotizables, pain thresholds have be increased with repeated hypnotic suggestions for hypnotic pain control strategies and patients need to be motivated to acquire specific skills training. At present, theoretical research links the effectiveness of hypnosis to conditioned learning (Holroyd, 1996).

Another specific therapeutic approach focusing on a stress reduction program in the treatment of 77 patients with FM has had positive results. Initial evaluations included a structured clinical interview; outcome measures included visual analogue scales to measure global well-being, pain, sleep, fatigue, and the experience of feeling refreshed in the morning. Patients also completed a medical symptom checklist, the SCL-90 (Revised), and measures of coping strategies, FM impact, and attitudes toward FM. Although the mean scores of all patients completing the program showed improvement, only the 51% who showed at least 25% improvement in 50% of the outcome measures were counted as improved (Kaplan, Goldenberg, & Galvin, 1993).

Perhaps the strongest new trend in psychological therapies for FM is family therapy (Nicassio & Radojevic, 1993). As shown in this chapter, there is no single psychological variable that can explain the discrepancy between physical symptoms of FM that are generally suggestive of mild to moderate medical disorders, yet which result in patient reports of chronic pain and suffering of disportionate magnitude associated with functional disability. Since no consistently universal psychological or (for that matter) physical etiology has been established, psychological treatment of individuals to correct psychopathological personality difficulties has not been as effective as initially anticipated. The focus in psychological therapies has thus concentrated more on helping patients develop more effective cognitive coping strategies. It is not surprising that treatment of FM patients is evolving toward family therapy approaches.

Pain-solicitous behavior has already received some attention in the family therapy literature. In pain-solicitous behavior, the spouse "encourages" pain by certain behaviors. Lousberg, Schmidt, and Goenman (1992) discovered that spouses who were identified as more solicitous had partners who reported an increase in pain, had poor endurance, and exerted less effort in physical activity. This finding is particularly relevant for therapy with FM patients, given the common pain complaints associated with muscle activity. Flor et al. (1989) also observed that the responses of significant others influenced pain impact ratings. Clearly, spousal responses have an effect on the extent to which a patient is able to cope with chronic pain. Three broad areas of dysfunction for FM patients as well as chronic pain patients generally who reportedly respond to family therapy have been identified: emotional distress, marital satisfaction, and sexual adjustment.

CONCLUSIONS

Chronic pain generally appears to reach its highest reported prevalence with a few diagnostic exceptions during middle age (Sternbach, 1986a) and is medically treated most intensively in this age group. The pain literature is extensive regarding psychological as well as medical treatment for chronic pain, especially back- and headache. Many other chronic pain syndromes as well have been systematically investigated in the research literature. However, FM is a chronic pain syndrome that is an exception in that it is gaining increasing acceptance and recognition in the medical community only in the last two decades as having a physiological basis rather than being a disorder of primarily psychological origin. As reported, this chronic pain syndrome affects approximately 2 to 5% of the North American population (Vaeroy, 1996; Wolfe et al., 1995). Understanding the medical etiology, progression, treatment, and degree of psychopathological comorbidity are still evolving regarding FM. Despite this uncertainty in theoretical perspective, there has been notable progress in treatment of this chronic pain syndrome both medically (Baumstark & Buckelew, 1992; Grassetto & Varotto, 1994) and psychologically (Holroyd, 1996).

Chronic pain in its various reported manifestations changes across age groups in terms of the epidemiology of diagnostic prevalence, patient demographics, and medical, psychological, and social etiology. The chronic pain syndrome of FM is relatively new as a medically reified pain syndrome and it provides a microcosm of the process of development of treatment strategies for chronic pain patients more generally.

CHAPTER 6

Transitional Issues during the Middle Years

Stress and Strain and Chronic Pain

Chronic pain has been described as a middle-age phenomenon. Onset of this condition(s) is often in the early 40s. The 40s transition has become a major topic of interest in research as well as popular literature. This is the period when women and men are said to leave youth behind and enter a new phase of life that is riddled with change, conflict, crisis, and often the first appearance of a variety of illnesses and the onset of aches and pain. This is also the time when people are said to become aware of their own mortality. The appearance of gray hair and a wider girth, menopause for women, sometimes declining libido in men, and loss of vigor are but very early reminders of ensuing old age.

On the family front, many changes become apparent. Children leave home, not infrequently women (mothers and wives) return to school and work, and couples are left to face each other without the buffering effect of children. These changes demand almost a redefinition of one's identity. Career issues, while still important, are more settled than during the earlier transitional phase and people generally have a sense of what may or may not be possible in terms of career.

In the ensuing pages we shall first explore the pertinent literature on the midlife transition, followed by life events experienced by chronic pain patients during this phase. We also shall examine the literature on illness and depression and illness during midlife, as well as family problems of middle-aged chronic pain patients. The rationale for doing so is based on the recognition that chronic pain patients are often depressed, either as a consequence of pain and loss or comorbidity, with family conflicts.

THEORIES OF MIDLIFE TRANSITION

The body of literature on midlife is enormous, and numerous books and articles exist on this topic. A debate concerns the actual period of time that spans midlife. For the purpose of our discussion of midlife transition, we shall confine ourselves to age 40 to 50 years, in accordance with Levinson's (1978) study. Our consideration of this topic will of necessity be modest, and we shall focus on what might be considered key transitional issues.

There is now wide consensus among scholars that midlife transitional problems are almost inevitable, and only the trials and tribulations of adolescence are in some measure comparable to this transition. Among the many writers, Neugarten (1968) recognized the significance of this transition. She recognized the changes in family roles during this period, the most prominent being reversal of the roles between aging parents and middle-aged adult children. This could also be the beginning of grandparenthood. A most intriguing phenomenon, she noted, was a shift in thinking about the future that translates into time left to live, which is a recognition of one's own mortality. She was emphatic that events associated with the midlife transition were in themselves not noxious and a vast majority of people completed this transition without the benefit of an existential crisis.

Levinson (1978) had a somewhat different perspective on the question of crisis associated with midlife transition. He investigated the phenomenon of midlife in a group of 40 men in their 30s and 40s. This study must rank as one of the most influential in terms of its breath and depth. Levinson made a number of startling findings, one of which was that this particular phase of life could not be completed without the benefit of a crisis. Crisis is not so much an event as it is a redefinition of one's identity, combined with the knowledge of mortality. For middle-aged men, this mortality also signifies the death of one's youth. Levinson goes as far as to say that "indeed, the person who goes through this period with minimal discomfort may be denying that life must change, for better or worse" (p. 26). However, he is cautious to note that this crisis is not necessarily pathological.

Levinson examined this transition from three discrete perspectives: (1) changes in biological and psychological functioning, (2) the sequence of generations, and (3) the evolution of careers and enterprises. We shall briefly discuss each of these perspectives. As much as biological and psychological changes occur throughout the entire lifespan, Levinson noted that reduced energy manifests in mostly minor ways during midlife. One is unable perhaps to sustain previous levels of hard physical work or sports, and a reduction in libido and energy are not unusual accompaniments of this stage. He points out, however, that these declines are not inevitable and many persons in this life stage maintain their earlier levels of functioning. Furthermore, it is more than feasible, he claims, that only a nominal decline during this phase may have the effect of enriching a man's life by shaking off the minor vanities, animosities, and envies of early adulthood.

Of particular interest from our view is Levinson's observation about biological declines during midlife. He noted that a man of 40, unless afflicted by illness, did not fall significantly below his optimal level of physical vigor. Nevertheless, the appearance of baldness, wrinkles, and paunch to most men herald the loss of youth and the imminence of middle age, although, as Levinson is careful to state, these changes are often of a cosmetic nature. His contention is that while bodily decline is generally slow and occurs almost imperceptibly, the cumulative effect of these changes can be significant. His views of middle adulthood are clearly pessimistic when he states that "for [a] large number of men, life in the middle years is a process of gradual or rapid stagnation, of alienation from the world and from the self" (p. 26).

In his discussion of the sequence of generation, Levinson's contention is that by the time a man attains age 40, he is more likely to be perceived by others as a parent than an older sibling. This change in perception is often a cause for dismay and depression and is one of the contributory factors in the struggle of changing identity for people in their 40s. Drawing on Erikson's (1960) concept of generativity versus stagnation, which coincides with Levinson's age range of midlife, he argued that development is a process in which opposite extremes are to some degree reconciled and integrated. To know and to experience stagnation, that is, being static, without hope or prospect, and perhaps most important, without a promising future is a prerequisite to generativity. The struggle to emerge from this enormous sense of isolation and self-doubt, another ingredient of crisis during midlife, is an integral part of the midlife transition. This recognition of vulnerability in due course becomes a source of wisdom, empathy, and compassion for others.

The final aspect of midlife transition relates to a man's careers in work, family, social settings, and future goals. The critical element here is his capacity to come to terms with his career and begin to accept his altered role in relation to his family and society at large. Even men with successful careers develop a sense of stagnation as their achievements are associated with the past. Levinson gives the example of Bertrand Russell, the famed English philosopher, who transformed himself from being purely an intellectual to a philosopher–politician–popular writer–moralist and more. This evolution, Levinson contends, and not any specific achievement, lies at the heart of development.

Levinson's contribution can be summed up in the following way. He divided the age 40 transition into two halves: 40 to 45 and 45 to 50. On the basis of his observations, he was able to delineate clearly three major areas of change and conflict that challenge men during the latter half of the midlife transition. This phase was characterized by a need for redefinition of one's self. Crisis, not in a conventional or clinical sense, was innate in this phase of development. Yet, the net effect of this transition was very positive, from self-preoccupation to concern for others, from careerism to mentorship.

Levinson's study was in the tradition of a sociological–anthropological paradigm. Empiricism was not the basis of his work. In recent years, some empirical literature has emerged. Some address Levinson's propositions directly and others indirectly. One study, directly relevant to Levinson's midlife issues in relation to women (Roberts & Newton, 1987) based on an analysis of four unpublished dissertations, confirmed that women and men progress through roughly the same developmental stages, and life stage specific tasks were also found to be similar. Beyond that, however, the way women worked on the tasks was rather different as were the outcomes. The authors explained these differences on the basis of the greater complexity of women's dreams and the problems encountered in living them out.

A different picture was presented by Hedlund and Ebersole (1983) in their findings of midlife transition issues. They interviewed 156 subjects, both men and women, divided into three age groups (35–39, 41–46, and 48–53), to explore their evaluation of midlife transition. Midlife transition failed to emerge as a significant period of reevaluation and the preoccupations were not significantly different than those of the other groups. They concluded that Levinson's key proposition that midlife was a period of the reevaluation of one's dream and one's meaning of life empirically could not be substantiated. On the other hand, important life events seemed to be of great significance in the reevaluation of midlife transition.

A more recent study of men's well-being at midlife found in a group of 75 middle-aged professional men that well-being was highly dependent on the quality of interpersonal relationships (Julian, McKendry, & McKelvey, 1992). The best predictors of men's well-being at midlife were perceived closeness to children, perceived closeness to wife, adjustment to the husband role, and number of close friends. These last two studies point in the direction that the midlife transition in itself is not perilous, but important life events combined with family conflicts and lack of social support could contribute to difficulties during this transition. Crisis, in the way of finding and accepting a new identity, which is at the heart of Levinson's idea, is not inevitable.

The other major contributor to our collective understanding of transitional issues is provided by George Vaillant (1977), in his Grant Study at Harvard University. This study followed 95 Harvard students who graduated during 1942, 1943, and 1944. They were followed up 10 years later and then again 20 years later by Valliant. This study involved a privileged section of American society, and yet some general conclusions pertaining to life transition issues appeared to have wider implication. Any single event in childhood, however noxious, did not seem to have any lasting effect on the person. Vaillant put it this way: "the quality of the whole journey is seldom changed by a single turning" (p. 368).

At age 47, when the grant study men were asked to review their lives, one telling finding was that most of them outgrew the crassness and the narrowness of the career consolidation phase (age 30 transition). One man, who was very ambitious at age 31, declared at age 47 that what he enjoyed most was watching others become more fruitful in their jobs; he worked hard to improve his company's performance and to win the affection of his shop steward. In other words, having achieved rather modest success for himself, he invested his efforts in being altruistic and cultivating meaningful relationships.

Vaillant concluded that normally occurring life stage events rarely precipitated a crisis. They were, by and large, anticipated events and people prepared themselves for their eventuality. Nevertheless, crisis could be precipitated by sudden events, especially if such events were not appropriate to that life stage. This is a rather different perspective than that of Levinson, whose contention was that crisis constituted an integral part of midlife transition.

Over the years, a certain amount of literature related to midlife crisis has emerged; we shall examine, albeit briefly, that body of literature. First, there does not seem to be consensus on midlife as being a crisis. Even among the three protagonists of midlife, only Levinson subscribes to the idea of crisis being inevitable as well as desirable for a successful completion of midlife transition. Vaillant and Neugarten differed in their understanding of this transition and did not regard crisis as inevitable.

A literature search revealed approximately 30 articles over the past 25 years dealing with midlife crisis. There was some evidence that specific events triggered crisis rather than existential concerns, or alternatively, midlife issues triggered events that led to crisis (Arnold & McKenry, 1986; Coche & Coche, 1986; Waskell & Owens, 1991). Arnold and McKenry (1986) investigated divorce as a phenomenon of midlife transition. Their subjects consisted of 13 men (aged 46 years) and 15 women (aged 44.7 years) who were participants in a divorce support group. The conclusion of the study was that midlife issues played a major role in the divorce, and also that spouses's midlife transitions were weighed more heavily than the subjects' own midlife transitions in judgments concerning causes of divorce.

Waskell and Owens (1991) investigated 376 adults (aged 30 to 60) to determine how they viewed their transitional issues between the ages of mid-30s and late 40s. The majority of subjects were enrolled in university programs; 260 identified that either they were in the midst of a crisis or had a crisis during that phase; 152 were able to identify the trigger event. Most of these events were either in the category of "change in self" or "work related." One is existential and the other environmental. This and the previous study seem to suggest that midlife issues can be triggered by issues and events, both internal and external.

However, Levinson's concept of midlife crisis, with some modifications, was supported by a few reports (Ciernia, 1985; Gutman, 1976; Oles, 1994). Of these, Ciernis's report of a group of businessmen between the ages of 30 and 60 years provided clear evidence that an existential concern, namely death, was at the heart of their midlife crisis. In a multicultural study of men, Gutman (1976) found that for the urbanized man the midlife issues were associated and often complicated by problems such as a liberated middle-aged wife, possible alcoholism, and the emergence of psychosomatic problems. The most remarkable finding of this complex study was that psychological changes during midlife transcended cultural differences.

Others, however, failed to find strong evidence to support this proposition (Brim, 1976; Costa et al., 1986; Gordino, 1983; Yagill, 1991). In a study of 206 Israeli women, Yagill (1991) found no evidence of midlife crisis. It must be noted, however, that the subjects were in their 30s, and as such did not meet Levinson's criteria of midlife. Costa et al. (1986) conducted a cross-sectional study of data from 10,063 32- to 88-year-old subjects to determine personality changes over time. His conclusions were that older subjects were slightly lower in neuroticism, extroversion, and openness; that age trends were curvilinear; and that there were no differences in personality scores that might be attributable to midlife crisis or transition.

The weight of the evidence, however, points in the direction that midlife is problematic. It is indeed characterized by many changes both internally and in the external environment. Life events during this phase have the capacity, as with all other life stages barring perhaps infancy and very early childhood, to give rise to crisis for individuals. Yet, there is little direct support for Levinson's radical notion that midlife transition could not be successfully completed without crisis.

LIFE EVENTS AND THE MIDDLE-AGED CHRONIC PAIN PATIENT

Midlife is associated with the emergence of many health problems. Risk factors of coronary heart disease (CHD) in middle-aged persons, for example, has come under the scrutiny of researchers (Falger, 1983; Peter, 1995), as has depression (Gallo, Royal, & Anthony, 1993), employment and depression in middle-aged women (Bromberger & Matthews, 1994), alcoholism and suicide (Roy, 1993), changes in hypothalamic–pituitary–adrenal axis function during midlife (Maes, Calabrese, Lee, & Meltzer, 1994), grief due to parental death (Moss, Moss, Rubenstein, & Resch, 1993), and problem drinking (Brennan & Moos, 1990).

For our purpose, the relevance of midlife issues in the lives of our mostly middle-aged patients in pain clinics is important. It might be instructive to review the kind of life events generally reported by these patients, and whether they are in any way related to midlife issues. Most of the articles on the topic of chronic pain and life events appeared between 1974 and 1997. Several papers were for a pediatric population (Alvarez & Dodge, 1990; Hodges et al., 1984; Walker et al., 1994). The rest could be divided into papers on chronic low-back pain (Atkinson, Slater, Grant, & Patterson, 1988; Feuerstein, Sult, & Houle, 1985; Naidoo & Pillay, 1994; Smith, Follick, & Ahem, 1985), temporomandibular pain (Marbach, Lennon, & Dohrenwend, 1988; Lennon, Dohrenwend, Zaruta, & Marbach, 1990), myofascial pain (Zaruta, Marbach, & Raphael, 1995), psoriatic arthritic pain (Gentill & Francescangaeli, 1987), headache (deBenedittis & Lorenzetti, 1992), and mixed pain groups (Egle, 1992; Pilowsky & Bassett, 1982).

A major problem of relating this literature to midlife transition is that the age range of subjects in general do not strictly conform to midlife. Several studies covered a wide age range, from early to late adulthood (ages 18 to 60+) (Atkinson et al., 1988; deBenedittis & Lorenzeti, 1992). It is impossible to determine the specific life stressors that confronted the populations during midlife. Others did not provide age-related information (Feuerstien et al., 1985; Zaruta et al., 1995), or the population was younger than midlife age range (Naidoo & Pillay, 1994).

One study that investigated risk factors for temporomandibular pain reported the ages of the cases as 38.0 years (SD = 11.7) and for the control group as 39.9 (SD = 11.5) (Marbach et al., 1988). Cases and controls did not differ in total number of life events. Nevertheless, events involving physical illness and injury strongly differentiated cases from controls. Midlife often marks the beginning of many aches and pains, depression, and a variety of other conditions. In the section that follows, we shall examine that literature. Another paper failed to find any relationship between stressful life events and pain, but did find an association between stressful life events and greater distress in a study of 110 myofascial pain patients (Zaruta et al., 1995).

The mean age of chronic low-back patients in a study that investigated life events was 41.0 years (Smith et al., 1985). Univariate correlations supported the prediction that high levels of negative life events were associated with high levels of several aspects of emotional distress. Negative events were associated with discouragement, depressed mood, dissatisfaction, anger, and social maladjustment. It is noteworthy that pain itself was seemingly unaffected by life events. On the other hand, it can be argued that the overall clinical picture of chronic low-back patients is immensely complicated by negative life events. This paper failed to furnish any information on the exact type and nature of life events.

This body of literature was somewhat disappointing from several perspectives. First, very limited information related to the nature of life events and their relevance to midlife could be deduced. Second, the age ranges of subjects were not directly relevant to our discussion of midlife transition. Third, life events as an etiologic factor in chronic pain was not categorically addressed. Rather, psychological outcome of negative life events was the focus of several studies. On the basis of these studies, it is almost impossible to make any claims of the etiologic significance of negative life events in the genesis of chronic pain of midlife onset.

A Case

While the significance of life events in the genesis of chronic pain or psychological distress due to chronic pain remains somewhat moot, the following case will help illustrate the vast number of changes precipitated by the emergence of chronic pain and disability in a 42-year-old man. From a clinical point of view, life events precipitated by chronic pain, while regularly observed in clinical practice, remain an underresearched area. This is the story of Mr. Magri, who, with high hopes, had immigrated to Canada from Europe some years earlier.

From all accounts he had realized the immigrant's dream. He found a well-paying job, bought a house and a car, and was well on his way to leading a good life. He was married with three children. His world came crashing around him following a work-related accident that damaged his hip and legs. The injuries were judged to be of a minor nature, and it was thought to be no more than a short-lived inconvenience. As with so many chronic pain sufferers, this uneventful beginning of his pain culminated in rendering Mr. Magri an invalid in 12 short months. His pain worsened to the point that he was unable to perform at work and lost his job. He received worker's compensation and began his search for a medical cure. Even in this short vignette, major events are apparent. He lost his job, a major undesirable event by any measure, a direct consequence of which was reduced income, which precipitated a major strain on family finances.

Mr. Magri's age is of some significance. He was just emerging from his age-30 transition and moving into a more stable occupational and family situation. As an immigrant, his view of himself was that of a successful man who had, so to speak, "arrived." Job loss to Mr. Magri and being on "charity," as he perceived the worker's compensation, caused him to almost completely lose his self-confidence. He embarked on a rather destructive course that culminated in suicide. His major complaint was that life had been unfair. He stated on more than one occasion that he had reached a stage in his life, following many years of struggle, when he deserved peace and tranquility. Prior to the accident, his life was almost idyllic. At times, he had difficulty in believing his good fortune. All that was taken away as a result of what was seen by all as a minor accident. We shall return to this case presently to discuss the impact of Mr. Magri's disability on his family. Two major events, a minor accident, which turned out to be not so minor, and job loss, ultimately cost this man's life.

Another aspect of Mr. Magri's behavior deserves attention. Having achieved and lost his position in society, he turned his attention to fellow sufferers. He devoted a great deal of time and energy to creating a peer support group comprising chronic pain sufferers. This group, with his leadership, started lobbying governments, health care services, workers' compensation, and other organizations to be more understanding of the plight of chronic pain patients. This aspect of his behavior could be viewed as the emergence of the altruistic aspect of him, which tends to make its appearance during the midlife transition. This case is indeed poignant from the view of demonstrating crisis. His crisis is not a perfect fit for Levinson's view of transitional or existential crisis. Rather, it confirms that events during midlife may have special significance, such as job loss and the emergence of health problems. The latter perhaps only accentuates the concerns about physical vulnerability and mortality. Job loss during this period assumes great significance, as alternative employment becomes less feasible.

Depression in Midlife

In this section we shall examine the relevant literature to determine if midlife heralds the beginning of depression. In the context of chronic pain, depression assumes a very special significance, as this condition is ubiquitous in the chronic pain population. Depression in the general middle-aged population has been the subject of investigation from several perspectives.

El-Rufaie and Absood (1993) investigated the prevalence, nature, and severity of depression in 217 Arab subjects, aged 16 and older. The total prevalence rate of depression was 27.6%. The morbidity rate was higher among women than men, but the population in the age range of 35 to 54 was the most susceptible to depression and anxiety–depression. The overall severity was in the mild-to-moderate range. This paper did not offer any theory to explain the high morbidity in the middle-aged group. Another study, however, offered a biochemical explanation for age variation in depressive illnesses (Maes et al., 1994). In a study of 118 patients with major depression and 80 controls, they found a major negative correlation between age and plasma morning cortisol in control subjects, but not in the depressed group. They concluded that middle age could be the turning point in hypothalamic–pituitary–adrenal axis function of normal versus major depressive persons.

Another study investigated the relationship between employment status of middle-aged women and depression (Bromberger & Matthews, 1994). This study involving 524 women found that nonemployed women reported higher levels of depressive symptoms than employed women, with nonemployed women with less education, low support from family and friends, and low marital satisfaction being the most symptomatic. It was found that new paid work had a beneficial effect on the mood of middle-aged women.

A study involving 102 middle-aged women investigated the impact of their mother's death (Moss et al., 1993). The sudden death of mothers caused more intense grief, less acceptance, and more thoughts of reunion than with deaths that occurred in nursing homes. This study measured depression, grief, somatic symptoms, impact on the sense of self, degree of acceptance of the death, and the quality of ties with the mother. The findings were complex, as many of these reactions were intercorrelated. Yet, they were differentially associated with characteristics of the daughter, mother, and the quality of their relationship.

Yet another investigation involving women aged between the early 40s and the early 50s reported that normative personality changes in these women were not interrupted by menopausal status, "empty nest" syndrome, or involvement in caring for parents (Helson & Wink, 1992). Around age 40, however, many women experienced turmoil. This study is important in supporting the view that from a psychological perspective, middle age is not necessarily a period of increased vulnerability for psychological distress.

In a very different kind of study, Gallo and colleagues (1993) studied the risk factors for the onset of depression in middle age and later life. All subjects with a history of major depression were excluded. In this epidemiological study of subjects 40 years and older, there were 180 incident cases and 960 subjects at risk for future occurrence of major depression. Risk of depression for those who were employed was not significantly different than for those who were not employed. On the other hand, those who had 12 years of schooling were at less risk for depression than less those who did not complete high school.

This brief incursion into the midlife–depression literature point in the direction that the evidence is equivocal. Depression may occur and the reasons may be biochemical or grief or significant demographic factors. Yet, there is also evidence that this phase may not be specifically vulnerable to depressive disorders.

The presence of chronic pain, however, seems to alter this lack of vulnerability to a substantial degree. The literature on pain and depression is of a magnitude to deserve a major review. Several such reviews were conducted during the 1980s, and the general conclusion was that while depression was not uncommon in patients with idiopathic chronic pain, it was not inevitable. There was a major shift away from equating chronic pain without organic cause with depressive disorders. Three facts emerged: first, that a proportion of chronic pain patients also suffered from major depression; second, that negative life events and financial hardship in conjunction with unremitting pain caused many patients to become sad and discouraged; and third, many patients with chronic pain were not depressed, although many of their symptoms such as low energy, low libido, and sleep disturbance overlapped with symptoms of depression.

It would be erroneous, however, to suppose that the debate is over. A quick glance at the most recent literature continues to be contradictory and confusing. Ruolf (1996) claimed that 50% of chronic pain sufferers also suffer from depression as comorbidity. His claim goes further to suggest that both depression and chronic pain share common biological pathways. Aggressive treatment with the new generation of antidepressants is strongly recommended. Eisendrath (1885) noted that many chronic pain conditions were associated with known psychiatric disorders such as somatization disorder, hypochondriasis, factitious physical illnesses, and pain associated with psychosocial problems. Here, we have two alternate, yet overlapping views of depression and psychiatric problems and chronic pain. One claims common biological pathways, the other claims chronic pain to be a primary psychiatric disorder. They are, of course, not mutually exclusive.

McGuigan (1995), on the other hand, found that psychosocial

factors were involved in the depression of chronic pain sufferers. Banks and Kerns (1996), in their extensive review of the pain and depression literature, concluded that the unique experience of living with chronic pain may account for the high prevalence of depression.

Overestimation of depression was recognized in a Finnish study, in which the researchers concluded that a diagnosis of depression based on a sum score of an inventory that contains somatic–vegetative signs of depression (inventories on depression almost always include somatic–vegetative signs) may lead to an overestimation of depression (Estlander, Takala, & Verkasalo, 1995). Even this short incursion into the current literature suggests unresolved diagnostic issues. This debate is likely to continue until such time that more objective laboratory-based investigation for major depression becomes available.

However, from a practical and clinical point of view, all the perspectives are important. Social and biological factors interact in complex ways to engender depression. Sometimes, one has primacy over the other. Treatment also has to be multidimensional. Perhaps a brief visit with the case of Mr. Magri may be useful to appreciate the complexity surrounding depression. Mr. Magri's pain was not altogether explicable on the basis of physical pathology, and the question of a psychiatric "overlay" was considered. He presented many of the common neurovegetative symptoms shared by chronic pain and depressed patients. As is so common with chronic pain patients, he was placed on 100 mg amitriptyline, which failed to produce the desirable change in his pain or mood. The dosage was varied, again without much benefit to the patient. His mood of anger on the one hand and overpowering feelings of dejection on the other could only be explained by addressing the monumental changes in his life, all precipitated by his accident and subsequent pain. An abbreviated list of those changes would include job loss, loss of income, loss of face to his friends and relatives, loss of purpose, loss of workmates, loss of position and authority within his family, and emerging behavioral problems with his teenage children (we shall elaborate on the latter in the next section). The fact that this patient's past history as well as family history of depression was negative is also noteworthy.

It is in relation to the management of Mr. Magri that the question of depression assumes special significance. In addition to an antidepressant, which had only minimal effect on his depression or pain, and other methods of pain management, considerable effort was invested in dealing with his precarious psychological state and his deteriorating family situation. Nothing proved particularly efficacious, and at the end Mr. Magri killed himself. The centrality of job loss loomed large in his case. Mr. Magri came from another continent to earn a living. Having attained his dream, to lose it all was more than was acceptable to him. Once he reached the judgment that his pain was not likely to become tolerable to the point that he could resume his normal living, he failed to see any purpose in his struggle. This case is instructive for the reason that as depression is viewed more often as an organic disorder, the prescribed treatment for which is medication, there is a danger of neglecting serious psychosocial problems that may be not only complicating the diagnostic issues but also adding to the risk of important matters being ignored.

Family Functioning

Family functioning of chronic pain patients is a relatively well-studied subject, and the following chapter is devoted to an examination of the role of family members in reinforcing pain behaviors. This section explores the kind of problems and conflicts experienced by pain patients and their families. First, we shall review briefly the more recent literature on family functioning, following by a family assessment Mr. Magri.

Investigation of family functioning of chronic pain sufferers began in earnest in the early 1980s. Much of the early literature focused on the impact of chronic pain on the spouse. This broadened into a general examination of family functioning from a systemic point of view. We shall examine the literature published during the 1990s.

The review articles on family functioning for chronic pain patients, all conducted during the 1980s, were unanimous in their recognition of family dysfunction caused by the presence of a chronic pain patient in a family system (Flor, Turk, & Rudy, 1987; Payne & Norfleet, 1986; Roy, 1982). These early studies continue to find support in more recent reports. In an important Finnish study involving 63 chronic low-back patients, Saarijarvi (1991) reported on the effectiveness of couples therapy. Patients were randomly assigned to therapy group and control group. At the termination of therapy, the treatment group showed significant improvement in communication, while communication had worsened in the control group. The Marital Questionnaire was derived from the Dyadic Adjustment Scale. In addition, six items were derived from the Marital Communication Inventory. Unfortunately, the authors did not provide any of the scores derived from these scales. Their conclusion was that couples therapy contributed to a better quality of life by improving communication. It would be reasonable to assume that these couples were faced with serious enough relationship problems to agree to couples therapy.

Extensive family problems were reported by a group of headache patients, and their problems were found to be far more serious than a control group without chronic pain (Basolo-Kunzer, Diamond, Maliszewski, Weyerman, & Reed, 1991). The authors compared 117 patient–spouse couples with 108 couples without chronic pain. The Family Adaptability and Cohesion Scale (FACES III) and Dyadic Adjustment Scale were used to assess family and couple function. Marital satisfaction was measured by marital satisfaction subscale of ENRICH. The findings in relation to family cohesion and adaptability were mixed. Mainly, the headache couples and controls were similar on these dimensions. Only five headache couples were found to be in the extreme range of family cohesion and adaptability, thus revealing chaos among these couples. However, the headache sample had twice as many extreme or seriously troubled families as balanced families. The overall findings were complex. Headache couples reported greater differences in consensus, cohesion, affection, and sexual relationships than did control couples.

There were also some curious findings. Patients with continuous pain were more likely to report greater marital adjustment than patients with episodic pain. This was perhaps an indication of adjustment and learning to live with pain, rather than coping with the uncertainty of intermittent pain episodes. Another finding of a paradoxical nature was that headache patients' severity of pain correlated positively with greater marital satisfaction. Perhaps this was an indication of pain eliciting affection and support (discussed in detail in the next chapter).

Thomas, Roy, and Cook (1991) reported on the family functioning in a group of college students and their parents with headaches and back pain. They used the Family Assessment Measure to assess family functioning. Much of the pain in this nonclinical population was in the mild-to-very-moderate range. Yet, serious family dysfunction was reported by these families. In the areas of communication, involvement, control, and values. The authors speculated that the high level of dysfunction in these families could not be accounted for by low-level pain in the subjects. Rather, the life stage of the family (fathers' mean age 45 and mothers' 36), in the midst of many changes, was the probable cause for family disruption.

The final study in this section reported on the differences between headache and back pain patients in their family functioning (Kopp, Richter, Rainer, Kopp-Wilfling, et al., 1995). In this pilot study, the family environment of 36 families comprising 154 individuals was investigated. The Family Environment Scale and Family Climate Scale were used to assess family function. Families of mothers suffering from headaches were compared with mothers suffering from back pain and a pain-free group of mothers. Each group comprised 12 families.

Intrafamilial expressiveness was a greater problem for the families with mothers with headaches compared to both comparison groups. In headache families, expression of feelings was constrained, combined with less spontaneity and a reluctance to express annoyance or criticism. On the positive side, headache families, in comparison to pain-free families, were better organized. These families demonstrated a sense of order, planning, and clear assignment of responsibilities. Again, the picture was mixed and complicated. In short, on some dimensions of family functioning the headache families had problems and on others they were more effective.

This brief update on the family function of chronic pain patients reveals a rather complex picture. While family functioning is often a casualty of chronic pain, many families continue to function at an effective level. There is little research to explain how and why such families are successful in maintaining their functioning. Perhaps future research could address that question.

Family Functioning of Mr. Magri

Following the loss of his employment and an almost complete lack of progress with treatment, he slowly began the process of slipping into the inevitable chronic sick role. Vast and unfortunate changes occurred in his family. He began to neglect his family responsibilities, lost interest in sex, which is commonly observed in this population, and consumed a large quantity of tranquilizers and narcotic analgesics. He became impatient with his children, being very short and irritable with them. He would undertake tasks he could not complete, such as painting the house or fixing his trailer. This further confirmed his state of disability, contributing to his increasing sense of uselessness. He was a traditional, authoritarian father and husband with rigid views on masculine roles that he could no longer successfully complete. These changes in Mr. Magri had an enormous impact on the entire family.

The family consisted of Mark, aged 18, Mary, aged 15, and John, aged 14, and Mrs. Magri, aged 43. They were faced with a multitude of problems. The children felt that they had lost a friend and a guide in their father. Most of the time he was unreasonable, demanding, and impossible to please. Mark and Mary were barely coping and John had turned to hard drugs.

Mrs. Magri's roles were drastically changed. She viewed her husband as ill and in constant need of medical care. She was vociferous about the failure of the medical profession to help her husband. On the domestic front, she had to assume responsibility for family finances, attend to the children's concerns, and frequently assume a mediating role between her husband and the children. Mr. Magri had been a policeman in his native country and had believed in strict discipline, which included physical punishment for the children. At the same time, he was a caring father and used to spend many hours playing with the children when they were young. He was genuinely fond of them, and despite his strict ways, all three children acknowledged that he was kind and considerate and that they could always turn to him for counsel and guidance. Since the accident, however, he was not only irritable and angry, but he seemed to be actively searching for ways to criticize them. He would ask one of the children to do a chore, criticize the child for not doing it well, and undertake it himself, the consequence of which was usually more pain and frustration. This pattern would repeat itself over and over.

The children found ways to stay out of Mrs. Magri's way: Mark busied himself with school work and stayed away from home as much as he could; Mary became tearful and depressed, her school work suffering considerably; and John found solace in drugs. Mr. Magri agreed during a family session that the children's complaints were justified, but he felt helpless to alter the situation.

Mrs. Magri's position was no less precarious. She had to cope with a worsened financial situation, a drug-addicted son, and a depressed daughter. She sympathized with her husband, but was unable to show any anger or openly to disagree with him. When it was pointed out that Mr. Magri had never made an effort to explain his conduct to the family, he acknowledged that he felt emasculated and that his anger and frustration was a response to the feeling. He often felt guilty for blaming the children, but failed to express his positive feelings. Being critical was the only avenue open to him for exerting his authority, but he was beginning to sense that they were all drifting away from him. He did not wish to behave this way, but he could not help himself.

This case was carefully assessed using the McMaster Model of Family Functioning. Space does not permit a detailed account of the assessment, but suffice it to say that pervasive problems were found virtually in every dimension of family functioning. In general terms, this case raises a fundamental question: When does a medical problem become a family problem? More often than not, with chronic pain, these problems grow slowly and almost imperceptibly. Initially, there is hope that a medical cure will be effected. Gradually this optimism gives way to anger and frustration and a gradual recognition that a cure may not be at hand.

Repercussions of this on the family may not be immediately apparent, because the family views the patient in a normal sick role. However, as the problems persist and the patient fails to recover and assume his or her normal roles, tensions mount and questions about the patient's health status begin to be hesitantly and then forcefully raised. The doctors may conclude that nothing is wrong with the patient. But if so, why does he or she act so strange? Is he or she mentally ill? These are some of the unasked questions by the family members.

SUMMARY

This chapter has presented an overview of the theories of midlife transition, and has attempted to relate some of the midlife issues to the middle-aged chronic pain population. Since the age of inception for pain clinic patients is about 42 years, midlife issues are indeed important from a clinical point of view. Depression, life events, family conflict, and intrapsychic and existential conflicts could be colored by the midlife transition of these patients, and the midlife issues could be of major significance in understanding the patient's response to pain.

CHAPTER 7

Families of Chronic Pain Patients

Help or Hindrance?

INTRODUCTION

In this chapter we shall attempt to address the family issues of middle-aged chronic pain sufferers from three diverse perspectives. Hopefully, these three perspectives will provide a more thorough answer to the question posed in the title. The three perspectives are: (1) the impact of chronic pain on the family system; (2) the role of the family as a source of social support; and (3) the family, or more specifically, the role of the spouse as a hindrance to the patient's recovery and well-being. The main thesis of this chapter is that any one of these dimensions alone is likely to distort the clinical significance of the very complex nature of patient–family interaction, as well as the negative and positive aspects of family as a central source of social support.

IMPACT OF CHRONIC PAIN

A great body of research literature has evolved over the past 20 years on this topic. The main conclusion of much of this literature is that the overall impact of chronic pain in family member has serious implications for the well-being of the family as a system, the children, and the spouse.

Chronic Pain and the Family

A respectable body of empirical literature has evolved over the past several years to show that virtually every measurable aspect of family functioning is affected negatively by chronic pain. Yet, the literature specifically dealing with the impact of chronic pain from a systemic perspective remains relatively small. It is the latter that will be briefly reviewed here. Clinical or case reports are excluded from this consideration and only research reports are included. It should be noted that the systemic view of the family reveals the functional as well as the dysfunctional components of the family as a whole. This perspective is important to adequately answer the question posed in this chapter, namely, the value of family support. If chronic pain families are at the dysfunctional end of the spectrum, the argument that the family is more of a hindrance than help gains added power.

Some of the early and pioneering work was conducted by a group at the University of Philadelphia Child Guidance Center. One of their studies found a relationship between certain family characteristics, such as overinvolvement, enmeshment, overprotective concerns, and failure to resolve conflict, and the exacerbation of pediatric abdominal pain (Liebman, Honig, & Berger, 1976). Unfortunately, the study was less than satisfactory from a methodological perspective due to small sample size, lack of a control group, and virtual absence of statistical analyses. It was also concerned with pediatric pain. This study is important, however, because family dynamics were implicated in the exacerbation and maintenance of chronic pain. The remainder of the literature involves chronic pain patients in their middle years and their families.

One of the earlier studies to investigate family and marital relationship and chronic pain was reported by Hudgens (1979). She investigated the functioning of 24 couples where one partner had chronic pain. Six areas of family functioning were investigated and were found wanting. Marital problems have been shown to be endemic in this population (Ahern, Adams, & Follick, 1985; Feurstein et al., 1985; Mohamed, Weisz, & Waring, 1979; Kerns & Turk, 1984). It should be noted that these studies investigated some aspects of marital relationships rather than overall family functioning, especially from a systemic perspective.

One of the early studies to do so was reported by Roy (1989). The study was based on detailed and systematic interviews with families. He conducted a comprehensive analyses of family functioning of 12 chronic back pain and 20 headache patients and their families. The McMaster Model of Family Functioning (MMFF) (Epstein, Bishop, Ryan, Miller, & Keitner, 1983) was used to assess these families. MMFF assesses the following dimensions of family functioning: (1) problem solving, (2) communication, (3) roles, (4) affective responsiveness, (5) affective involvement, and (6) behavior control. Families in both groups were found to be deficient almost in all areas of functioning.

Problem solving was problematic for 75% and 100% for back pain and headache families, respectively; communication was at the pathological end of the continuum for 50% of back pain and 75% of headache families. Problems related to various aspects of role function were endemic in both groups. Nurturance- and support-type roles were ineffective for 75% of back pain and 100% of headache families. Marital and sexual gratification was lacking for 75% of back pain and 60% of headache groups. Occupational and household roles were compromised for 50% of back pain and virtually none of the headache group.

Almost 65% in both groups expressed difficulty in affective responsiveness, which assesses the family's capacity to express appropriately a wide range of emotions. Affective involvement, which is concerned with relationships between family members, was found wanting in 83% and 60% of back and head pain families, respectively. Finally, behavior control, which examines the rules by which families conduct their lives, was seriously flawed in 83% and 80% of back and head pain families, respectively.

This clinical study, even without the benefit of a control group, revealed enormous problems in family functioning in two of the most common groups of patients seen in pain clinic settings. Most of these families were troubled and functioned at the low end of family functioning. To seek confirmation of these clinical findings, a carefully designed study was implemented (Roy & Thomas, 1989; Thomas & Roy, 1989).

Fifty-one consecutive patients, who were referred by their physicians to a pain clinic located in a teaching hospital, were the subjects for this study (Roy & Thomas, 1989). These patients were typically referred for their intractable pain. The subjects completed a comprehensive demographic and pain questionnaire, the Beck Depression Inventory (BDI) and Family Adaptability and Cohesion Scale (FACES III), Couple Version. FACES measures two dimensions—family cohesion and family adaptability—and derives 16 specific and three general types of families, namely, balanced, mid-range, and extreme. Statistical analyses comprised χ^2, *t*-tests, and discriminant function analyses. The first two tests are recommended by the proponents of FACES as the most appropriate.

In terms of overall family functioning, marital discord was quite common and the families were functioning in the mid to extreme ranges. These families evidenced more difficulties in the area of family adaptability than in family cohesion, which in effect demonstrated their inability to adapt to or cope with the altered circumstances brought on by chronic pain, among other factors. On family cohesion, the families were functioning in the borderline of being connected. Spouses assumed the central task of keeping the family together, which contributed to a somewhat better state of family cohesion. This study lends further credence to the notion that families and couples with chronic pain tend to show a high level of family dysfunction.

In a subsequent analyses, nine clinically depressed subjects from the above group were compared with 42 nondepressed patients. Depression in conjunction with pain significantly affected family stability (Thomas & Roy, 1989).

Findings of the previous study mainly were negated in an investigation of family functioning in a group of headache patients and a control group (Basolo-Kunzer et al., 1991). In this controlled study, 117 headache patients were compared with 108 married couples for marital and family functioning. FACES III was used to assess family cohesion and adaptability. They tested a series of hypotheses, with mixed outcome. The most critical for the purpose of this chapter was that contrary to prediction, no significant differences emerged between the two groups on family cohesion, adaptability, protection, or satisfaction. Only five headache couples were in the dysfunctional range on adaptability and cohesion.

One plausible explanation for the seeming contradictory findings of this study with that of Roy and Thomas (1989) is that major differences were found in the clinical populations in the two studies. There were the age differences, headache subjects' mean age was 40 years and the Roy and Thomas study population was nearly 49 years. Also, the headache patients, despite differences in frequency and intensity, represented a more homogeneous group than a mixed group of chronic pain patients comprising back pain and an assortment of other chronic conditions. It was more than likely that the headache group was more functional than the mixed chronic pain patients in the Roy and Thomas study. This observation is partly supported by the fact that only five couples were in the extreme range on the adaptability scale, whereas discord in the area of family adaptability was quite prominent in the Roy and Thomas study.

A more important observation is that there is much risk in lumping together many and varied kinds of chronic pain conditions under the rubric of chronic pain. As was observed earlier (Roy, 1989), families with headache compared to backache patients tend to be more functional and not as drastically affected in their marital relations.

Two more recent studies also produced contradictory findings (Nicassio & Radojevic, 1993; Naidoo & Pillay, 1994). In a comparative study of 44 rheumatoid arthritic patients (mean age, 55 years) and 46 patients with fibromyalgia (mean age, 51 years), Nicassio and Radojevic (1993) reported that, on the basis of the Family Environment Scale, the scores of the two patients groups were similar to the scores for the normative sample. The patterns of scores were reflective of families in both groups being supportive and as promoting a high degree of independent behavior in their members. These families, in other words, were mainly similar to normal families.

Even the authors were surprised by their findings and they offered the following explanation. It is quoted in full to convey some of the misgivings expressed by them: "The lack of empirical work on the nature of family functioning in these illness groups makes it difficult to interpret the positive characteristics portrayed by the subjects in this research" (Nicassio & Radojevic, 1993, p. 315). They speculated that the "halo" effect in conjunction with the fact that these subjects were volunteers, well-educated, and knowledgeable about their illness could have influenced the outcome. To ameliorate the problem, they proposed detailed questioning via interviews to minimize the risk of responses being in the socially desirable.

Naidoo and Pillay (1994) compared 15 women, aged 30 to 35 years, with chronic low-back pain with 15 healthy controls. On the Cohesion, Expressiveness, and Conflict subscales, which measure the relationship dimensions, of the Family Environment Scale, significant differences were found on cohesion, conflict, independence, and organization. The pain group was significantly compromised in its overall family functioning. Other than reiterating this finding, the authors did not speculate or offer any reasons for this. This finding was in the expected direction and the data simply confirmed it.

Taken together, these studies present a confusing picture. It will be somewhat perilous to claim that family functioning is invariably affected adversely by chronic pain, especially when the methodological issues often identified in the literature remain unresolved. Different populations, different instruments to measure family function, different analyses, and different sampling techniques would suggest that any effort to bring some order to this body of literature may not be productive and each study ought to be judged on its own merit.

Impact on the Children

Common sense suggests that parental illness, especially of a chronic nature, may indeed produce negative health and emotional consequences for the children. Yet, the evidence is far from certain. In an extensive review on this subject, Roy (1990–91) posed two questions: (1) What might be the prevalence of physical, emotional, and psychiatric problems in the children of medically ill parents compared to the general population? (2) What might be the risk factors that predispose the children of the medically ill parents to psychological and medical vulnerabilities? The first question could not be answered due to major methodological shortcomings in most of the studies and the second question received only partial answers. Severity of the illness and the gender of the sick parent received partial validation as predictive of vulnerability. Yet, even the severity question was ambiguous. The major conclusion was that a good deal was unknown in this important field of health research. There is, of course, much evidence of the adverse effects of parental mental illness on children.

Direct evidence for any relationship between parental chronic pain and negative health effects on children is just emerging and the conclusions are at best tentative (Chun, Turner, & Romano, 1993; Dura & Beck, 1988; Mikail & von Bayer, 1990; Raphael, Dohrenwend, & Marbach, 1990; Rickard, 1988; Roy et al., 1994). A brief review of the literature is presented. While the literature addresses complex issues, it is virtually impossible to derive any conclusions on the prevalence of psychosocial problems in the children of pain sufferers.

Dura and Beck (1988) examined many aspects of family functioning of children living with parents with chronic pain, diabetes, and healthy parents. Each group consisted of seven mothers and seven children. Children with mothers with chronic pain were more psychologically disturbed than the comparison groups and their family functioning was also more compromised than the comparison groups. A noteworthy point about this study is that while the children of mothers with chronic pain were significantly more depressed than the two comparison groups, all three groups scored well below the clinical range on the depression scale.

A more recent study also investigated school adjustment and emotional health of 29 children of 29 parents with chronic pain and a control group (Chun et al., 1993). Children of fathers with chronic pain were significantly less socially competent than children of female patients. Overall, children of pain patients had significantly more behavior problems and were less socially competent than the control group, although a low prevalence of psychopathology was found in both groups.

Roy and colleagues (1994) investigated the health and well-being of 31 children of 19 patients attending a pain clinic. Only three children, less than 10%, were found to be vulnerable on objective psychological measures. The family profile of these three children was also at variance with the other children in the sample. The negative effects of parental pain on children was far from pervasive. There was no control group in this study. However, within-group comparisons were carried out between the children who gave evidence of difficulties and those who did not. The sample size was another limitation. However, the findings of this particular study were in the opposite direction to the previous two studies.

Three studies examined the specific pain disorders of severe headaches (Mikail & von Bayer, 1990) and temporomandibular (TMJ) pain (Raphael et al., 1990) in parents and assessed their negative impact on the children and children of chronic low-back pain (Rickard, 1988). In their comparison of children of parents with a control group, they concluded that the children of headache sufferers were more somatically focused, had more headaches, and showed greater maladjustment and lowered social skills than the control group (Mikail & von Bayer, 1990). A major problem with this study was the number of *t*-tests conducted; not surprisingly, a low level of significance was found on many of the associations.

Raphael et al. (1990) compared children of 31 patients with TMJ with 47 controls. Children of TMJ parents reported significantly more illnesses and accidents. They offered a variety of plausible explanations for their findings. Rickard (1988) compared 21 children with parents with chronic low-back pain, 21 children with diabetic parents, and 21 controls. The study concluded that the children of parents with chronic low-back pain were significantly more external than the other two groups on the health locus of control. Teachers of these children also reported a significantly higher frequency of complaints, crying, whining, avoidance behaviors, dependency behavior, absenteeism, and visits to the school nurse than all other children in the study.

A preliminary conclusion to be drawn from the above review is that the negative effects of parental pain on children are not inevitable. Studies that examined well-defined clinical populations found a stronger relationship between the two. With less well-defined diagnostic groups, the findings were ambiguous.

Impact on the Spouse

The topic of depression and distress in the spouse of the chronic pain patients has come under periodic scrutiny. Some of the early investigators reported a higher prevalence of depression in these spouses than in control groups (Kerns & Turk, 1984; Mohamed et al., 1979; Shanfield, Heiman, Cope, & Jones, 1978). More recent studies have confirmed that finding and have gone beyond the question of depression alone (Flor, Turk, & Scholz, 1987; Romano, Turner, & Clancy, 1989; Saarjarvi, Hyppa, Lehtinen, & Alanen, 1990; Schwartz, Slater, Birchler, & Atkinson, 1991). Three of these latter studies involve chronic low-back pain patients and their spouses. The findings of these studies are briefly discussed.

Although these four studies vary in scope and details they agree on the deleterious effects of chronic pain on the spouses' health and well-being. Flor and colleagues (1987), in a study of 58 chronic pain patients and a diabetic control group and their spouses, found a number of interesting associations. Considerable pain-related changes were noted in marital satisfaction, health and mood of the spouse, and sexual relations. The main conclusion of the study was that chronic pain could have wide-ranging detrimental consequences for the spouses of chronic pain patients.

Romano and colleagues (1989) also reached similar conclusions in a study of 83 chronic low-back pain patients (41 men and 42 women) and their spouses. They investigated the level of physical and psychosocial disability, pain behavior, marital satisfaction, depression, and pain severity. Interesting gender-based differences emerged. Some of the characteristics were more evident in male patient couples rather than female patients and their spouses. Spouses of male patients reported significantly lower marital satisfaction than did their partners, spousal marital satisfaction decreased with increased depression in the patient, and greater spouse depression was associated with greater depression and lower marital satisfaction in patients. Spouses of male patients reported higher levels of depression than the spouses of female patients and were found to be the more vulnerable of the two groups. For reasons not altogether self-evident, spouses of male patients were more vulnerable than the spouses of female patients. The authors offered a number of plausible explanations.

Another study involving 63 chronic low-back pain patients (31 men and 32 women) found chronic low-back pain patients and spouses expressed high marital satisfaction (Saarjarvi, Hyppa, Lehlinen, & Alanen, 1990). Female spouses, however, reported significantly more musculoskeletal symptoms during the past week than their male counterparts and there was some suggestion that female spouses experienced more somatization than male spouses. Their conclusions was that chronic low-back pain causes psychological distress in the spouses and that spouses should be included in the treatment of the patients.

Schwartz and colleagues (1991) investigated impact of chronic low-back pain in 29 patients and their spouses. Twenty-eight percent of the spouses were depressed based on the BDI. Depressive symptoms were noted even in patients with moderate levels of pain. Subsequent analyses of the data revealed that spousal depressed mood could be predicted by patient's average pain, patient's reported levels of anger and hostility, and the spouse's level of martial satisfaction. The clinical implication of these findings were discussed.

These four studies and a plethora of previous studies point in the direction that spouses of chronic pain patients become vulnerable and are an "at risk" group for a variety of health problems, primarily depression. Yet, it must be noted that while a proportion of spouses fall prey to ill health, many, if not most, do not. They continue to cope in some manner.

In this context, the study of Rowat and Knafl (1985) is important. They explored the social factors underlying the distress experienced by the spouses of chronic pain patients. They investigated a convenience sample of 40 spouses (21 men and 19 women) whose partners were attending a pain clinic with a variety of chronic pain complaints. Spouses registered a total of 123 health concerns—emotional, physical, and social.

The spouses were divided into two groups of high distress and low distress. Distress was defined as the number of areas of life altered directly as a result of pain. Twelve spouses, 10 of whom were female, were identified as high distress. In addition to the health-related problem, they reported changes in four or more out of seven dimensions of family life. These dimensions were relationship with children, marital partner, and friends; division of labor; decision making; family activities; and financial management. Uncertainty emerged as a major source of anxiety in the spouses. They were uncertain about the pain and family life. This study provided powerful evidence that for a segment of spouses of chronic pain patients the emotional, social, and health cost is very high.

To summarize, despite depression and distress in the spouses of chronic pain patients, many continue to function well and remain a source of emotional support for their partners. In the following section, the social support literature is examined.

SOCIAL SUPPORT

In the previous pages, the question of overall family functioning and impact of chronic pain on children and spouses was considered to raise the possibility that families may be so impaired by this affliction in a member or as a family that their capacity for support would be severely compromised. The evidence is mixed. Many families become dysfunctional to varying degrees. Not many children seem to suffer, but evidence suggests that many spouses fall prey to depression and distress. Yet, many families adapt and cope with their altered circumstances.

In this section, more direct evidence will be sought for the question: Is the family for a chronic pain patient a source of support or not? Does the relevant literature illuminate or confuse the question? The review that follows purports to shed some light.

The family can be a source of problems and also a source of support for the pain patient. Perhaps there is no inherent contradiction in that proposition, since not all families fall prey to the negative effects of chronic pain. To complicate the matter further, there is some evidence to show that in healthy marital relationships, the well spouse is likely to engage in pain-reinforcing behaviors, thus counteracting any likely benefits of treatment. It is noteworthy that this proposition runs counter to a substantial body of evidence that strong marital relations act as a powerful buffer against morbidity.

It must be noted that the general social support literature is enormous, but there is considerable agreement about the positive functions of social support and its protective powers. This particular review will focus only on the role of family support for the chronic pain patient. While the amount of relevant literature is by no means large, it is substantial enough to merit a review.

Social Support and Chronic Pain Literature

In a review of this nature, an important consideration must be the very concept of "social support" and how this concept was defined and measured. While, on the surface, the general tenor of the research literature finds much support for a positive relationship between the availability of family support and low levels of pain, high levels of functioning, and other measures of positive outcome, yet these findings bear close scrutiny of the research methods employed in these studies? Another issue already alluded to is the plethora of outcome measures employed in these studies. Rather varied yardsticks are used to measure outcome. Then there is a body of literature, mainly in behavioral medicine, that purports to show the negative role of the spouses in reinforcing pain behaviors. This review will first examine the body of research that mainly showed the benefits of family support in coping with chronic pain; second, the studies with contrary findings; and finally an overview of the current state of knowledge in this field will be examined.

Benefits of Social Support

Weickgenant, Slater, and Patterson (1993), in their investigation of coping activities of patients with chronic low-back pain, made a critical observation. Disinclination to seek social support in the face of exacerbation of back pain was a factor that added to the general level of stress of the patients. This point is frequently overlooked in the literature. Pain and depression are prescriptions for social isolation and not uncommonly are observed in clinical practice. Availability of social support must be separated from utilization of such support.

The role of the "supportive" spouses in mitigating depression in chronic pain patients was reported over a decade ago by Kerns and Turk (1984). Since then, the positive role of the family members in the lives of chronic pain patients has been explored from various perspectives. In a more recent study, Goldberg, Kerns, and Rosenberg (1993) found further support for the role of the spouse in buffering 105 chronic pain patients against depression. Level of support was measured by the Support Scale from the West Haven–Yale Multidimensional Pain Inventory (WHYMPI) measures of patients' perceptions of the amount of supportiveness and attentiveness provided by their spouses to their pain problem. Findings of this study were of a complex nature, but the basic hypothesis of the role of social support, in this instance spousal support, in the amelioration of depression was confirmed.

Jamison and Virts (1990) compared 233 chronic pain patients who described their family as supportive with 275 age-matched chronic pain subjects with a self-report of family disharmony. On all measures of illness behavior and level of functioning, the group with supportive family relationships was significantly better functioning than the group without such support. Perceived family support was found to be positively correlated to less illness behavior and better coping.

In a 1-year follow-up of the completion of pain treatment, a random sample 181 subjects completed a set of questionnaires to determine the effects of family support or lack thereof. Predictably, patients reporting high level of family support reported significantly less pain intensity, less reliance on pain medication, and a higher level of activity. Patients with nonsupportive families relied on medication, reported more pain sites, and used more pain descriptors to describe pain. These patients were also more emotionally distressed and engaged in inappropriate pain behaviors.

Several points are noteworthy in this study. First, as the authors noted, family support was strictly determined by patients' perception of such support. In the absence of a valid measure of social support, sole reliance on patient's perception is somewhat limiting. Perception may be at variance with reality. Another point is lack of information on the families. This was an important omission. Composition of families, family functioning (pre- and posttreatment), and the identity of the caregivers (or sources of support within the family) are critical determinants of social support and the investigators ignored all of them. Many of the criticisms apply in various degrees to this entire body of literature.

Jamison and Virt's (1990) finding supported an earlier study by Manne and Zautra (1989) who, in an investigation of the role of support for a group of patients with rheumatoid arthritis, found that patients who perceived their spouses as supportive engaged in more adaptive coping. An interesting aspect of this finding was that spousal criticisms in themselves had no effect on the subjects' perception of supportiveness. Gaston-Johansson, Gustaffson, Felldin, and Sanne (1990), in a controlled study of fibromyalgia and rheumatoid arthritic patients, concluded that social support provided by significant others played a part in decreasing stress and facilitating effective coping. An important finding of this study was that neither of the groups received much support in the area of protection from psychological exertion. The implication is that the nature and quality of support are important determinants of their protective functions.

The importance of some of the family variables were discussed by Benjamin et al. (1992). They examined knowledge and beliefs of 34 family members about chronic pain patients. The findings were discouraging and a cause of concern to health care providers. Most caregivers subscribed to the organic view of pain and expressed much dissatisfaction with the up to date investigations to determine the causes of pain. They felt uninformed about many aspects of the patients' problems. The authors noted that "many appeared to hold strongly inappropriate views." On the positive side, nearly one third of the subjects thought that psychological factors were important. The authors concluded that with proper information and education, family members could have facilitated psychological treatment. This was a pilot study with a small sample size and focused on physical aspects of treatment. Despite these limitations, this study lent credence to the merit of involving family members in the management of the patient.

The final study to be considered in this section was conducted by Faucett and Levine (1991) in which they measured the impact of social network on pain complaints in patients with arthritic and myofascial pain disorders. Their conclusion was that generalized conflict with the entire social network was more harmful for patients with myofascial disorders in terms of their affective pain than patients with arthritic disorders. They noted that the cumulative social network stress rather than conflict with intimates was associated with increasing pain in the myofascial pain group, which identified pain as more wretched, tiring, fearful, sickening, and punishing. This study is important for two reasons. First, it examined the consequences of a stressful social environment. Second, by doing so, it demonstrated the importance of looking beyond the intimate relationships. The conclusions clearly showed the necessity of creating a stress-free environment.

Negative Consequences

The most telling criticism about the limitation of family as a source of social support has come from an examination of the role of the spouse in pain-reinforcing behavior. In study after study, high marital satisfaction has been found to be positively correlated to negative pain reports and more manifest pain behaviors. In view of the vast literature on the topic of spousal pain-reinforcement behavior, only a selected review of the more complex studies are presented. These studies recognized the complexity underlying the simple equation that healthy marital relationships equal spousal reinforcement of pain behaviors. Conceptualization of pain behavior in these studies is strictly predicated on the principles of operant conditioning.

The most recent contribution to this debate has been that of Turk, Kerns, and Rosenberg (1992). Their review of the literature and a report of their own investigation led them to conclude that positive attention (support given by the spouse) correlates positively with pain and disability. Having made that claim, they described some of the limitations of such a simplistic conclusion. They made an interesting distinction between "positive" and "problematic" support. This may have important clinical implications for couples and marital therapy. However, the most problematic aspect of their report was the narrowness of the concept they employed to describe a complex phenomenon. There was some recognition of the limitations of their central assertion that "positive attention appears to be positively associated with pain and disability ..." (p. 261). That a complex marital relationship that was influenced by a whole host of factors could be reduced in rather simplistic terms of desirable and undesirable support fortunately did not escape their attention. Finally, their assertion that the social support literature was inclined to adopt a simplistic view of that concept was more a reflection of their desire to prove a point than an accurate assessment of the value of social support.

Turk was not alone, of course, in proposing a more complex understanding of the negative consequences of spousal support than some of his predecessors. Kerns, Haythornthwaite, Southwick and Giller (1990) came to similar conclusions and proposed a model of optimal marital interactions that includes positive communication and mutual reinforcement for desired behaviors and outcomes, but also ignores undesirable behaviors. The authors cautioned against drawing any firm conclusions from their study due to the correlational nature of the data.

Basolo-Kunzer and colleagues (1991) investigated the relationship between marital and family adjustment in 117 headache couples and 108 marital couples without headaches and concluded that patients with greater marital adjustment were more likely to have more continuous headaches than patients with less marital adjustment. This study was a departure from the operant conditioning approach, as the investigators employed Minuchin's (1974) psychosomatogenic model to investigate family dysfunction and any relationship between family dysfunction and head pain. A central problem in the methodology was that the instrument employed to investigate family functioning measured some of the attributes of Minuchin's model and not others. Furthermore, Minuchin's model was predicated on psychosomatic problems in children, the central feature of which was marital conflict.

Very little effort was made to explain the key findings of Bosolo-Kunzer et al. (1991), and the fact that greater marital adjustment correlated positively with continuous head pain was far from self-explanatory. Theoretically, this paper was poorly conceptualized and the findings, interesting as they were, were perplexing, as they tended to go against the central tenet in Minuchin's model which was that effective family functioning reduced the vulnerability of children to a variety of psychosomatic disorders.

Bradley, Richter, Scarinci, and Schan (1992) investigated, among other variables, the role of spousal or significant other's pain reinforcement behaviors in the self-reporting of pain in subjects with unexplained chest pain with subjects with other kinds of chronic pain complaints. Their conclusion was that the partners and spouses of patients with unexplained chest pain were more inclined to be solicitous, which, the authors presumed, led to high levels of verbal and motor pain behaviors from the chest pain patients.

DISCUSSION

A good marriage is bad for pain is the conclusion of many studies. The family support literature takes exactly the opposite view. The literature on family functioning, in part, confirms the deleterious consequences of chronic pain on family functioning.

In the event that a spouse is depressed and fails to take an active interest in or perhaps is even hostile to the patient, and thus does not engage in pain-reinforcing behavior, is the treatment outcome for pain more optimistic? Are pain-reinforcing behaviors and supportive family relations mutually exclusive? Does one counteract the negative or the beneficial effect(s) of the other? Answers to these questions are far from self-evident. Yet, the intrinsic value of social and family support as a buffer against stress, resulting in more effective coping with multiple vicissitudes of life, is not without power.

Another issue that has eluded the researchers is the complexity of marital relationships, again by adopting a strictly operant conditioning perspective, which at best is myopic, of what is defined as the pain-reinforcing behavior. That such behaviors exist is undeniable. Reasons for their presence in marital or family relations tend to be more complex than behaviorists acknowledge. Behaviors do not exist in a vacuum. They tend to serve multiple functions. If a spouse engages in reinforcement of pain behaviors out of care and concern (universally acknowledged by behaviorists), then simply educating the spouse that such behaviors are harmful for the person they care about can be relatively easily corrected. But anyone with even a rudimentary knowledge of family relations will be troubled by such a simplistic view of marital relations. An operant model of chronic pain that proposes the spousal reinforcement of pain behavior (usually a function of healthy marital relationship) contains all the problems of an extremely narrow view of human conduct to the exclusion of all else. That is its strength and its main limitation.

Roy (1985) argued that the very concept of spousal reinforcement of pain was narrow and myopic. This concept is the equivalent of a biomedical model that takes a narrow view of the disease and tends to disregard the individual with the disease, as though the disease occurs in a vacuum. The pain-reinforcement perspective suffers from the same deficiency. It disregards the complexity of family relationships and completely ignores the dynamics that underlie two persons' behavior toward each other by ignoring the reasons for such behavior.

An illustration of this is a spouse who actively promotes pain behavior in a patient to retain control of family finances. For the first time in their long marriage, a wife has gained control and is not willing to let go. This example is not far-fetched. In this hypothetical situation, the behaviorists are unlikely to eradicate the "undesirable" behavior of the wife without addressing the underlying conflict, which they are not likely to concern themselves with. Therein lies the major therapeutic deficiency of this proposition. In medicine, a doctor can prescribe insulin to control diabetes, but with a noncompliant patient this simple way of controlling the disease may assume extraordinary complexity. The patient's social and psychological issues must be addressed to promote collaboration. The same principle applies to understanding and effectively treating negative pain-reinforcement behaviors in the spouses.

Yet, the notion of positive and negative support is a meritorious pursuit. For any clinician engaged in family work with chronic pain patients, this distinction is a daily fact of life. Concern and worry on the part of a well-meaning spouse that the patient is perhaps doing too much and should be discouraged is not an uncommon complaint.

Despite the debate about whether or not family responses to pain are inherently reinforcers (Fordyce, 1993), Turk, Kerns, and Rosenberg (1991) have proposed a new approach to research as well as and, perhaps more important, provided some preliminary guidelines for practitioners to be more attentive to what may or may not be positive support. This perspective of support, despite its oversimplified operant view of negative support, that is, spousal reinforcement of pain behaviors, is perhaps the most important contribution to the debate and hopefully puts to rest the silliness of the all-or-nothing (in the sense that support is invariably positive or invariably negative) approach to investigating the complexity that surrounds the questions of spousal reinforcement of pain behaviors for sufferers of chronic pain. Perhaps the emphasis on family itself as either the repository of all ills or all good is at the heart of many misconceptions and the consequent narrowness of the scope of most of the investigations examined here.

PART IV

PAIN ISSUES AND THE ELDERLY

CHAPTER 8

Epidemiology of Chronic Pain in the Elderly

The definition of chronic pain for the elderly is the same as that used for all other age groups. Chronic pain is defined as any pain lasting longer than 3 months and not responsive to standard medical treatment, or "an unpleasant sensory and emotional experience associated with actual or potential tissue damage or described in terms of such damage" (International Association for the Study of Pain Subcommittee on Taxonomy, 1986, p. 246).

Aging does not inevitably result in declining health accompanied by chronic pain. Age and health status are relatively independent for an individual at any age, including the elderly. Furthermore, there is greater variability in the range of health status in the elderly than for any other age group. However, on a group basis for the elderly the inconvertible truth is that as the body ages, there are increases in the incidences of a number of painful diseases (Rowe & Besdine, 1982; Kwentus, Harkins, Lignon, & Silverman, 1985; Melding, 1991; Helme & Gibson, 1996). The elderly are also more at risk for chronic pain as a direct result of accidents, because injuries may not heal completely or may take a longer time to do so (Rubenstein, Robbins, & Josephson, 1991). It has even been hypothesized that the elderly who take psychotropic drugs are at increased risk of injury and pain. In the elderly, many of whom are prescribed psychotropic drugs, there is vulnerability to drug effects that may predispose some individuals to accidental injuries. There is an extensive body of data demonstrating psychomotor function impairment for benzodiazepines and antidepressants, which establishes a clear basis for risk between medication and accidents for the elderly (Higgit, 1992).

With increasing age, metabolic changes also occur that can impact the pain experience in the elderly. With aging, there are also changes in neurochemical levels that can produce medical conditions involving mental dysfunction. Some of the more common dysfunctional psychiatric disorders such as depression, anxiety, panic attacks, and dementia share comorbidity with pain complaints. In a review of epidemiological placebo-controlled, double-blind studies, it was shown that 15–33% of medical inpatients suffer from affective disorders compared to 2–4% of the general population. In these same studies, patients with one or more chronic medical illness also had a 41% increase in the relative risk of developing a psychiatric disorder (Katon & Sullivan, 1990).

Furthermore, since the elderly as a group are prone to medical illnesses, this results in high use of physician and self-prescribed medication. It becomes important then to recognize that the medications taken by the elderly including psychotropic and analgesics may impact on the prevalence of pain complaints (Jenike, 1996). This interaction between pain reports and medication is considered a significant factor and has been investigated in the literature. For example, in one large study the prevalence of multiple analgesic use for 1192 men and 2025 women (aged 65 years and older) was reviewed. Approximately 14% of the women and 10% of the men analgesic users reported taking multiple medications during the preceding 2 weeks. Men who had reported pain in the preceding year were most likely to be multiple analgesic users. As well, female multiple analgesic users were similarly characterized as reporting pain and having limited physical functioning and higher depressive symptoms (Chrischilles, Lemke, Wallace, & Drube, 1990). From the preceding discussion it is evident that there are a number of factors that impact on pain in the elderly. These factors include health status, risk for accidental injury, mental stability, and medication use.

Another important variable that can influence when a pain symptom is reported or instigates seeking medical treatment is the perception of the elderly as to the meaning of the pain symptom. One study investigated the reasons for physician consultation of 667 elderly people (aged 65 years and older) living in community settings. Results indicated that uncertainty regarding the potential seriousness of a pain symptom, level of pain severity and interference of activities, as well as causal attributions for the pain were the most consistent predictors of physician contact. It was concluded that patients did not respond to the symptom per se, but rather to their perception of the symptom and its effects on their lives (Stoller & Forster, 1994).

Chronic pain in its many manifestations has a high prevalence in the elderly, but this phenomenon is not a diagnostic artifact caused by different norms used in classifying pain as clinical or chronic in nature because of the age of the patient. For example, demographic, health, and psychological factors were examined for 361 patients (mean age 69.2 years) reporting osteoarthritis pain. Approximately 90% of the diagnoses were confirmed by evaluation by physicians (Cronan, Shaw, Gallagher, & Weisman, 1995).

Overall, the changes in the structure and function of bodily processes due to aging are specific rather than general. Research investigating pain in the elderly is increasing, but generally it is not a central topic in the medical literature. Rather, the focus of the medical literature is on specific diseases such as rheumatoid arthritis or osteoarthritis (Davis, Cortez, & Rubin, 1990; Ferrell et al., 1994), shoulder disorders (Chard, Hazleman, King, & Reiss, 1991), abdominal pain (Bugliosi, Meloy, & Vukov, 1990; Gibson & Helme, 1995), ischemic heart disease (Miller, Sheps, Bragdon, Herbst, & Dalton, 1990; Ambepitiya et al., 1994), myocardial infarction (Bayer, 1988), hip pain (Schon & Zuckerman, 1988), neck pain (Moskovich, 1988), and lung cancer (McCorkle et al., 1989) rather than pain per se. From the preceding, it could be surmised that chronic pain issues in the elderly are well researched. Yet, to place pain research with elderly populations into perspective "each year over 4000 papers (Medline data) are published on pain, but less than 1% of these focus on pain experience or syndromes in the elderly person" (Melding, 1991, p. 119; Jacox, Carr, & Payne, 1994).

DEMOGRAPHIC CONTEXT FOR THE ELDERLY WITH PAIN

In order to more meaningfully understand the epidemiology of chronic pain in the elderly, it is necessary to understand the physiological, psychological and social influences that form the context surrounding chronic pain reports. The elderly are increasing within the general population in North America at a rate exceeding all other age cohorts. In the 1990s, approximately 15% of the population will be 65 years or older, and by 2040 it is estimated that as much as 25% of the population of North America (90 million) will be in this age range (Guralnik, Yanagashita, & Schneider, 1988). Individuals in this age group are also increasing proportionally in the world population. In 1992, it was estimated that there were more than 342 million individuals older than age 65. This figure has been increasing by approximately one million a month (US Bureau of the Census, 1992). These increases are due to a number of factors such as: (1) improvements in medical technology, (2) new drug developments, (3) better education, (4) individuals leading healthier lifestyles, (5) decreased mortality rates of infants and mothers, (6) better control of infectious diseases, and (7) wider access to medical care. However, the increase in this population also means that chronic pain in the elderly will be a medical and psychological issue of mounting importance. Current projections for the average longevity in the United States and Canada from census data in the 1990s estimate 83 years for females and 79 years for males. These figures represent estimated averages, which means that generally for individuals reaching the age of 65, due to the mortality that has already occurred within their cohort, they can expect to be functional well into their 80s (Melding, 1991).

Gerontologists divide those over 65 into three groups: the young-old (65–74), the old-old (75–84), and the oldest-old (85+). The oldest-old group, which currently stands at approximately 1% of the general population, is projected to rise to 5% of the population by 2050.

Helme and Gibson (1996), in a major review, concluded that chronic pain in the elderly has a high overall prevalence associated with increasing chronic pain until a peak in the 60s (Brattberg et al., 1989; Andersson et al., 1994) followed by a decline in the 85+ cohort, which is the oldest-old category (Thomas & Roy, 1988a; Mobily et al., 1994). Another general feature of the demographics of aging is that women represent approximately 75% of the elderly population after age 75 (US Bureau of the Census, 1992). In elderly women pain complaints are the single-most common reason for seeking medical help (Andersson, 1994). Another interesting aspect of gender differences in the elderly that may affect the reporting of pain is difference in the level of social support available for the elderly female chronic pain sufferer. Approximately 80% of men between the ages of 65 and 74 are married compared to only 49% of the women (US Bureau of the Census, 1992).

PAIN PREVALENCE IN THE ELDERLY

In any consideration of the prevalence of chronic pain in the elderly, it is necessary to note that the pain literature is composed of different samples of the elderly population. The pain literature shows wide variability in the rate of prevalence, probably depending on whether the sample was drawn from the community, an institutional setting, pain clinics, or convenience samples. The research relating to the prevalence of various types of chronic pain in the elderly ranges widely from 22% (Crook et al., 1984) to 88% (Mobily et al., 1994). Overall, studies report pain in the community elderly population as very high. Demlo, Laing, and Eaton (1986) reported that approximately 80% of an elderly sample reported just rheumatic complaints alone. Other studies (Roy & Thomas, 1986; Thomas & Roy, 1988a; Mobily et al., 1994) found that over 80% of their elderly samples reported pain problems across combined pain sites. Sternbach (1986a) drew his sample of persons over 65 from the community, which constituted 16% of the total population from a national United States survey. He found: (1) 50% reported headaches, (2) 49% reported backaches, (3) 42% reported muscle pains, (4) 31% reported stomach pains, and (5) 71% reported joint pain in the past year. In yet another large study of 3097 of elderly individuals (aged 65+ years), approximately 86% reported pain of some type and 59% reported multiple pain complaints (Mobily et al., 1994). Joint pain was the most common site of reported pain, followed by night leg pain, back pain, and leg pain while walking. As reported severity of pain increased, there was a corresponding increase in negative impact on daily activities. These findings are consistent with those of Gibson and Helme (1995), who reported joint and abdominal pain as the most common pain sites in the elderly. In the elderly, frequent abdominal pain is a common source of chronic pain. It has been estimated that 11 of every 100 elderly experience abdominal pain, and of these difficulties 95% were chronic indigestion. Among the individuals sampled who had abdominal pain, chronic constipation and/or chronic diarrhea were also common, yet only 23% had seen a physician for pain in the prior year (Bugliosi et al., 1990).

Although aging per se is not the cause of pain, with increasing age the incidence of a number of painful diseases does increase with aging (Helme & Gibson, 1997; Melanson & Downe-Wamboldt, 1995). The elderly are more frequently diagnosed with vascular disease, neurological degenerative conditions, neuropathies of diabetes mellitus, malnutrition, Herpes zoster (or shingles), and cancer, and most commonly diagnosed with osteoarthritis, rheumatoid arthritis, osteoporosis, and osteomalacia (Rowe & Besdine, 1982; Kwentus et al., 1985; Melding, 1991). It appears that there is a clear positive association between chronic pain risk factors and aging based on measures of prevalence of serious diseases. In the institutionalized (nursing home) samples of the elderly, the range of reported pain prevalence is between 70 and 83% (Roy & Thomas, 1986; Ferrell et al., 1990; Parmelee, Katz, & Lawton, 1991; Sengstaken & King, 1993).

It is considerably less clear regarding the various relationships between chronic pain complaints in the elderly and (1) physical sensory threshold changes and aging, (2) psychological dysfunction and aging, and (3) comorbidity with painful medical conditions that increase with age. All these factors, however, have important implications for baseline expectations of chronic pain in the elderly and will be briefly examined.

SENSORY THRESHOLD SHIFTS FOR PAIN AND PREVALENCE IN THE ELDERLY

Based on a review of the literature, Harkins (1988) observed that a decline in sensitivity with many of the senses has been well documented. According to current research findings, starting as early as age 50 and typically by age 60 there are general decreases in visual acuity and a loss in the ability to perceive depth. There is a decrease in hearing sensitivity overall, and most notably the higher frequencies are the first to show loss of sensitivity. Sensitivity to taste and smell also shows a decline across aging that is notable; these changes are often accompanied by shifts in food preferences for individuals as the number of tastebuds decline (Murphy, 1982). In addition to the sensitivity declines in sensory thresholds already mentioned, there are also obvious changes in physical appearance with aging such as hair loss in men related to hormonal changes and stopped shoulders in women associated with loss of bone density. There are also decreases in reaction time, agility, physical mobility, and physical strength (Buskist & Gerbing, 1990).

However, the laboratory study of pain thresholds and pain perception in relation to aging at present has not produced evidence of the same consistent decline in sensitivity that has been found for other sensory thresholds (Gibson & Helme, 1995; Harkins & Price, 1997). Pain threshold can be, at least in theory, quantitatively measured in physical units, unlike pain tolerance, which can only be subjectively assessed. For example, cutaneous pain thresholds are believed to be lower in women than men and tend to increase with advancing age (Procacci, Bozza, & Buzzelli, 1970). Chakour, Gibson, Bradbaer, and Helme (1996) have suggested that differential age-related pain sensitivity to heat is mediated through the relationship between myelinated A-delta and unmyelinated C fibers. A-delta fibers were hypothesized to be responsible for sensory discriminative features of acute pain sensation, while C fibers were hypothesized to be associated with diffuse, dull, burning pain sensations.

Overall, there is typically small variation (under 20%) across time in pain thresholds in individuals, as well as minimal variation in pain threshold (under 30%) across the different areas of the body of an individual. Tucker, Andrew, Ogle, and Davison (1989) found a rapid rise in pain threshold until age 25, followed by a more gradual rise in pain threshold until about age 75. After age 80, the wide variability of pain thresholds did not allow general conclusions. Further, this study found no sex differences in pain threshold; also, it significantly found no differences in pain thresholds between patients with pain and subjects without pain.

In two older studies, Harkins and Chapman (1976, 1977) found no age differences in pain thresholds; however, they found that shock intensity was discriminated better by young adults than older adults. It is difficult because of different research designs as well as varied methodologies to evaluate whether these earlier results are in fact contrary to more recent findings.

Threshold is primarily a measure of the sensory dimension of pain. Current thinking conceptualizes pain as having multiple dimensions including psychological and social aspects. Pain tolerance, rather than pain threshold, is actually more relevant to pain reports in the elderly. A multidimensional etiologic model of pain views pain differently from heart rate or blood pressure in that pain cannot be measured directly. Pain assessment involves inferences of "pain" from self-reports and other pain behaviors (facial expressions, protective behaviors of painful area, etc.).

According to Fordyce (1983), all pain behavior can be caused either by a direct nociceptive stimuli or alternately because the pain behaviors have come under the control of learning or operant control. Thus, it is quite possible to have similar degrees of physical injury and yet have dramatically different reports of pain. Conversely, it is possible to have dissimilar degrees of physical injury and reports of pain that are essentially the same. Finally, Fordyce (1983) suggests that the similarity or differences in reported pain may be caused by a single or more likely multiple psychological and social moderator variables that may distort an accurate relationship between physical injury and pain.

A direct example of this phenomenon was shown in a study by Sorkin, Rudy, Hanlon, Turk, and Steig (1990), where the physical and psychosocial characteristics of elderly and younger chronic pain patients were compared. The elderly group had more frequent abnormal medical findings, yet there were no significant differences on measures of self-reported activity, pain severity, life interference, or emotional or worry reactions in response to pain. Perhaps this phenomenon is related to recent evidence suggesting that older adults tend to attribute many of their pain symptoms to old age (Cook & Thomas, 1994). The pain threshold perception in many older adults is further complicated because of the presence of multiple health problems with vague symptoms that can affect the same anatomical region (Barrows, 1995).

CHANGES IN THE PREVALENCE OF PAIN REPORTS AS A FUNCTION OF AGE COHORT

Epidemiological research on the relationship between reported pain and aging has found mixed outcomes as to the direction of the association between aging and reported pain (Gibson & Helme, 1995). They found that self-reported pain across common pain sites with the exception of joint pains appears to decline after age 65 in the elderly. This phenomenon is a reversal in the direction of the association between age and reported pain, as reported by Crook et al. (1984). In that study in a general population, it was found that 16% reported pain during the past 2 weeks. The reported pain increased with age, such that 25% of those aged 61–70, 29% of those aged 71–80, and 40% of those over 80 reported pain. These results are consistent with the public's general perception of the relationship between pain and aging. However, a number of studies have reported that when the elderly are compared with young and middle-aged populations, the elderly report less overall pain. Specifically, Harris (1985) found younger individuals report more headache, backache, muscle pain, stomach, and dental pain than the elderly. Only joint pain reports increased with advancing age. The Nuprine Report (Starback, 1986), using a large representative sample from the United States, and Thomas and Roy (1988b; Thomas, Roy, & Cook, 1992), using Canadian samples, all reported decreasing pain reports for headache, neck pain, backache, muscle, chest, and stomach pain with increasing age. Again, the major exception was increased reports of joint pain with increasing age. These latter findings are generally consistent with other studies reporting decreasing pain reports from middle age to seniors (Brattberg, Porter, & Thorslund, 1989; Andersson, 1994; Mobily et al., 1994).

There are several explanations that may help our understanding of this apparent contradiction in reported pain when comparing young adult cohorts with elderly cohorts. First, with aging there is an increase in the general population in prevalence of illnesses with pain as a primary symptom. This would suggest that the pain literature should then show increases in pain being reported by the elderly. This appears to be accurate only for joint pain, while for all the other common pain locations there seems to be the opposite phenomenon of decreasing pain reports with older age cohorts. However, the issue here may not be discrepancies in the prevalence of the actual existence of pain in the elderly but rather contradictions in the prevalence of "pain reporting." There are many pain problems in the elderly that are common and seriously distress an individual but are relatively brief in duration, and so may not be reported. Also, pains that may be present may not be reported by the elderly because of a longer lifespan perspective of stoicism and minimal reporting of pain that is not chronic (Gibson, Katz, Corran, & Farrell et al., 1994). Finally, pain of shorter duration may not be remembered or may not be present at the time that the pain research data collection took place.

One theoretical perspective that might help our understanding of the possible mediating variables that impact on pain-reporting behavior in the elderly is a peer-modeling social learning approach. Thomas and Roy (1988b), using this model, investigated familial and peer models as well as personal pain and illness experiences as mediating variables across the lifespan. Differences in attitudes and behaviors involving chronic pain were compared between elderly and young adults. It was found that the number of familial and peer pain models (with specific illness) were related to perceptions of vulnerability and worries regarding these same illnesses and subsequent reported frequencies of pain complaints. This study demonstrated one way in which the presence of social models affected attitudes, which in turn was related to pain reporting.

As noted earlier, health status among the elderly tends to vary greatly and any generalized assumptions about the health of the elderly must be made with caution. Roy and Thomas (1988a) compared two age cohorts of elderly. Pain was reported by 81% in the 60s group and only 64% in the 80s group. The pain and age relationship was nonsignificant, but demonstrated a strong trend for the older-elderly to report less pain than the younger-elderly. The main findings in this study were that the older-elderly did not show significantly more pain as a group compared to the younger-elderly. Actually, the older-elderly reported less chronic pain than a group in their 60s (64 to 81%), while reports of recent illness differed by only 1% between the two age groups. For the 60s group, 44% reported recent illness and 56% did not report illness within the past 6 months. With the 80s subjects, 45% reported a recent illness and 55% indicated no illness during the past 6 months. These findings would be generally consistent with those from Gibson and Helme (1996), since their conclusion was that the reporting of chronic pain decreases with age in the elderly after age 65.

There may be one exception to this phenomenon: a rise in pain reports in the elderly just prior to death. In a study by Moss, Lawton, and Glickman (1991), the pain reported in the year prior to death by 200 elderly people (mean age, 77.4 years) was investigated. In retrospective reports by a surviving family member or spouse, pain was rated as increasing during the last year of life, and 66% of the elderly sample reported more or less continuous pain during the last month of life.

Not only has approaching death been found to be associated with more reported pain in the elderly, but chronic pain in the elderly is also associated with increased risk of suicide and death anxiety. In one study, 178 homebound elderly people (aged 65.5–87.3 years) participated in an investigation of death and dying anxieties. Results found three major categories of elderly fears: (1) physical pain and suffering, (2) risk to personal safety, and (3) threat to self-esteem and the uncertainty of life beyond death (Fry, 1990). In another study, 139 individuals who had attempted suicide were interviewed; it was reported that 52% of them suffered from a somatic disease and 21% were on daily analgesics for pain. The individuals that suffered from a somatic disease differed from other people in the study on depression scores, age, pain, and the presence of psychosis. Fewer of the somatically ill had a psychosis. Individuals who complained of pain were more often depressed and abused medicine. The seven patients who later committed suicide were older and tended to have painful somatic diseases (Stenager, Stenager, & Jensen, 1994).

SUMMARY

In conclusion, there appear to be a number of factors that interact when attempting to understand the epidemiology of pain in the elderly. First, as an age cohort, the elderly are the fastest growing segment of the general population in North America. Women tend to live longer than men on average, so that the pain issue in the elderly is one that includes a gender focus. With increasing age there is also an increase in the prevalence of specific diseases (such as arthritis) that frequently include pain as a primary symptom. In addition to increased risk for many medical conditions—both physical and mental—having comorbidity with pain complaints, there is an interaction factor between medication use and pain reports. It cannot be stressed too strongly, however, that individually there is the widest variability of health status of any age cohort in the elderly age group. Aging per se at an individual level physiologically is not directly or indirectly linked to increased pain prevalence.

There appears to be uniformity in rates of acute pain reported across all age cohorts. However, between age cohorts of young adults and the elderly there appear to be differences in the reporting of chronic pain. The elderly, with the exception of joint pain, tend to report less chronic pain across common pain locations, which appears discrepant considering that the incidence of a variety of diseases increases among the aged. Yet it is noteworthy that empirical evidence shows that pain reports tend to decline with age. The mechanisms that govern this apparent paradoxical phenomena may be different for the old vis à vis young and the young-old vis à vis the oldest-old. The discrepancies in pain reporting between the young adult cohorts and elderly cohorts may be in part a function of different expectations. Young adults have the expectation of little or infrequent pain based on a general public perception of youth and good health being pain free. In previous chapters this illusion has been shown to be flawed. When a painful condition occurs for a younger person, however, it violates their expectation and they report the pain. In the elderly there is a longer perspective of pain based on lifespan experience with pain such that intermittent pain is viewed as normative and not reported unless more extensive criteria are met in regard to severity and duration.

Finally, there appears to be an association in the elderly between pain and fears of death and an actual relationship between death and pain in the year preceding death. At this time, the literature is not well developed, and it remains to be seen if in fact there is an epidemiological basis between increased pain prior to death in the elderly.

CHAPTER 9

Role of Psychopathology in Chronic Pain in the Elderly

As the body ages, a number of painful diseases begin to make their appearance (Rowe & Besdine, 1982; Kwentus et al., 1985; Melding, 1991). In addition, the elderly are more at risk from the long-term effects of accidents, which often take longer to heal and result in chronic pain (Rubenstein & Robbins, 1984). As a result, most studies tend to report rather high rates of incidence and prevalence of painful problems in the elderly. Demlo et al. (1986) reported that approximately 80% of an elderly sample reported rheumatic complaints alone. Other studies (Roy & Thomas, 1986; Thomas & Roy, 1988a; Mobily et al., 1994) found over 80% of their elderly samples reported pain problems across combined pain sites. Sternbach (1986a) reported on a sample of elderly subjects (age 65 and older), which constituted 16% of the total population from a national United States survey. He found that (1) 50% reported headaches, (2) 49% reported backaches, (3) 42% reported muscle pains, (4) 31% reported stomach pains, and (5) 71% reported joint pain in the past year. Clearly, chronic pain has a high prevalence in the elderly. A critical issue then becomes what is the role of psychopathology either in the etiology of or response to chronic pain in the elderly.

PSYCHOLOGICAL FACTORS IN CHRONIC PAIN AMONG THE ELDERLY

The significance of psychological factors in chronic pain varies across the adult lifespan. Epidemiological research on pain has shown that complaints of chronic pain are lower in the elderly, with a few specific exceptions (such as joint pain), than in younger age cohorts. This negative correlation between combined reports of chronic pain and advancing age, although not universal, is generally supported by the current pain literature (Harris et al., 1985; Sternbeck, 1986a; Thomas & Roy, 1988a; Thomas, 1993b; Mobily et al., 1994). Such a finding suggests the importance of psychological factors rather than physical as important determinates in the reporting of chronic pain, since health status on average is better for young adults than the elderly. The International Association for the Study of Pain (1986) defines pain as: "an unpleasant sensory and emotional experience associated with actual or potential tissue damage or described in terms of such damage" (p. 246), and makes no stipulation that pain in the elderly is qualitatively unusual. Therefore, prevalence differences between age cohorts are not due to definitional shifts.

In general terms, most chronic pain conditions in the elderly have an organic basis, and psychogenic pain is considered to be less common than in the younger population. Diagnosis of chronic pain conditions in the elderly requires the differentiation of nociceptive, neurogenic, and psychogenic pain influences. This diagnostic differentiation can be made more complicated in the elderly because sensorineural thresholds are altered and thermal sensation is often diminished (Hardy, 1995).

There are also metabolic changes that occur with increasing age that can be associated with common psychological disorders such as depression, psychosis, violence, agitation, anxiety, panic, obsessive–compulsive disorder, pain, and dementia. Neuropsychiatric disorders in the elderly, such as dementia, may occur alone or in combination with neurological or medical illness. Mental illnesses, although low compared to other age cohorts, are not uncommon in the elderly, and as the elderly population increases in size, so will the prevalence of these illnesses (Jenike, 1996).

Comparisons of combined psychiatric disorders (American Psychiatric Association, 1987) for different age cohorts found that persons over 65 had the lowest prevalence rates. However, the comorbidity between complaints of chronic pain and psychological factors such as depression and anxiety in the elderly is very common (Kramlinger, Swanson, & Maruta, 1983). According to the *Diagnostic Statistical Manual of Mental Disorders*, fourth edition (DSM-IV) (American Psychiatric Association, 1994), the prevalence of chronic pain complaints attributed to Pain Disorder Associated with Psychological Factors, and Pain Disorder Associated with both Psychological Factors and a General Medical Condition have an estimated annual prevalence rate of between 10 and 15%. The DSM-IV also indicates that females are inclined to report more headaches and musculoskeletal pain; however, the DSM-IV does not report on differences in prevalence by age for many common pain complaints.

SOMATIZATION DISORDER

Somatization Disorder has an estimated annual prevalence rate between 0.02 and 2%. Onset typically occurs before age 25, and is reported approximately ten times more frequently in females than males. Although Somatization Disorder may have an early onset according to DSM-IV, it still occurs with frequency in older individuals as well. Pribor, Smith, and Yutzy (1994), evaluating 353 adult women (aged 18–86 years) with pain problems, found a prevalence of 24% of the patients aged 55 years or older. However, the sample of older women did not differ from younger women in the proportion of those who had a somatization disorder, in the number of somatic symptoms, or the characteristics of their pain complaints.

Because somatization may overlap with medical illness, bereavement, and atypical presentations of depression in the elderly, there are difficulties in diagnosis that raise questions surrounding the age of the typical onset for somatization. However, if, as conventional medical belief suggests, onset of somatization typically occurs in youth, then this disorder would appear to be highly resistant to change when the primary symptom is chronic pain, since the sample of older women (Pribor et al., 1994) did not differ demographically from the younger women in number of surgeries or medical or psychiatric hospitalizations. One would expect that if onset of the disorder were at a younger age, then the number of hospitalizations for medical or mental reasons would have been greater for the older women than for the younger women. Therefore, the group of older women with Somatization Disorder reported in this study had onset when they were older or had onset of somatization in their youth and the disorder persisted unresolved into their later years with fewer hospitalizations than younger women with recent onset of the disorder.

HYPOCHONDRIASIS AND DELUSIONAL DISORDERS SOMATIC TYPE

In another category in the DSM-III relating to chronic pain complaints, Hypochondriasis and Delusional Disorders Somatic Type has an estimated annual prevalence rate between 4 and 9%, and is equally common in males and females. There was no information in the literature as to prevalence by age. In a study by Barsky (1993), hypochondriasis as a psychiatric disorder and its relationship to aging were examined. Barsky noted that the elderly were at especially high risk for certain factors likely to foster hypochondriacal symptoms including chronic pain. These included increasing medical morbidity and bodily decline, social isolation, and psychiatric disorders that commonly have hypochondriacal symptoms as secondary features. According to Barsky, because of the long-term psychological features of this disorder, the management of the elderly hypochondriacal patient is best conceptualized of as care, not cure. This approach would require a major shift in perspective from medical to psychological etiology, where the focus is on helping the older patient cope and endure their symptoms rather than trying to eliminate them or expect the symptoms to diminish or cease with medical treatment and time.

The perception in the general public and medical community is that chronic pain complaints in the elderly do not have a strong psychological factor. Such a view is understandable, since any pain complaint of primary psychological etiology in an elderly population likely has comorbidity with an actual physical dysfunction, injury, or disease process. Thus, chronic pain complaints are not typically viewed as independent of physical status and reported as psychological disorders. Furthermore, the observation that chronic pain in the elderly is infrequently hypothesized as associated with psychological dysfunctioning may also reflect the fact that less than 5% of all individuals aged 65 or older attend pain clinics. In addition, because of the difficulty in diagnosis of psychosomatic pain, such a diagnosis would be even less likely to occur outside of a pain clinic where physicians experienced with hypochondriasis in the elderly are most likely to practice. Another point of note is that evidence suggests that altered physiology of pain mechanisms combined with psychological attitudes, such as stoicism and reluctance to confirm the presence of pain, may functionally raise the pain threshold psychologically, but this situation would not necessarily result in a formal diagnosis of psychopathology (Gibson et al., 1994).

DEPRESSION AND CHRONIC PAIN IN THE ELDERLY

In an epidemiological survey on pain and depression of 1319 men and 1704 women (aged 25–74 years) in the United States, 14.4% of the individuals reported chronic pain related to the joints and musculoskeletal system. Approximately 18% of the individuals reporting chronic pain also had depression; this was in contrast to 8% of individuals who did not report chronic pain. Depressive symptoms were more evident in women than in men (Magni, Caldieron, Rigatti, & Merskey, 1990).

The relationship between chronic pain and depression has been repeatedly found in the literature looking at the elderly (Roy et al., 1984; Parmelee, Katz, & Lawton, 1989; Sullivan, Turner, & Romano, 1991; Katz, Parmelee, & Stream, 1995; Hodgkiss, 1997). The relationship between pain and depression is complex both psychologically and physiologically. From the psychological perspective, Turk, Okifuji, and Scharff (1995) reported on a cognitive–behavioral mediation model to aid in explaining the association between pain and depressed affect in the elderly. This view suggests that cognitive appraisal variables have a mediating effect on the pain–depression relationship. Support for this position was drawn from a strong direct association between pain severity and depression that was observed in the older but not the younger patients. It should also be noted that the cognitive processes occurring during depression have been found to be similar to the cognitive processes when experiencing pain (Peterson & Seligman, 1984).

A psychological explanation between chronic pain and depression is also supported by another study where it was found that functional disability (but not physical illness) accounted for differences in reported pain between nondepressed individuals and those tending toward clinical depression (Williamson & Schulz, 1992). Because functional disability mediated the relationship between pain and depressed affect, as well as between illness and depressed affect, Williamson and Schulz suggested that both pain and functional disability were psychological factors influencing expression of symptoms of depression.

One psychological explanation for the relationship between pain and depression in the elderly hypothesizes that depression may psychologically sensitize individuals to the point that their psychological reactions to physical discomfort become intensified to pain sensation (Waddell, 1987). Waddell even argues that the physical stimulus that triggers a painful sensation may across time become less salient, and emotional distress such as depression becomes responsible for sustaining the psychological experience of pain. Whatever the mechanism, depression appears to have a strong association with chronic pain in the elderly, but the causal direction of the relationship has not been consistently demonstrated.

Presence of pain symptoms in clinical depression is relatively common not only in the elderly, but for all ages. Conversely, chronic pain patients not infrequently develop some form of depressive disorder. This finding may be in part due to symptoms common for both disorders (e.g., disturbed sleep, anxiety) that are prominent among both pain patients and depressed patients. Where pain–depression comorbidity exists, it appears that susceptibility to both dysphoric physical symptoms (including pain) and psychological symptoms (including depression) interact to exacerbate both conditions (Von Korff & Simon, 1996).

In addition to psychological explanations for the comorbidity of pain and depression there are also biological explanations. One such explanation describes how selective serotonin reuptake inhibitors, including fluoxetine, fluvoxamine, citalopram, paroxetine, and sertraline, may be mechanisms through which pain and depression are linked at a neurochemical level. The literature clearly supports the role of reuptake inhibitors in some conditions of major depression. Data concerning their role in other conditions such as panic disorder, premenstrual tension, chronic pain, dementia, and personality disorders with aggressive or impulsive features are preliminary but promising. The variety of clinical uses for these substances may compel reexamination of traditional diagnostic categories and theories of how antidepressants work (Boyer, 1992). Another hypothesis involving a neurochemical link between pain and depression that has been explored is that medications prescribed to treat symptoms of chronic health problems including chronic pain in the elderly frequently can aggravate a subclinical depression already present or cause mood reactions similar to depression. Some examples are antihypertensive medications, which cause depression in 20% of adults taking them, as well as hormones, corticosteroids, or antiparkinsonian drugs (Klerman, 1983).

GENDER, PAIN, AND DEPRESSION IN THE ELDERLY

In a study by Parmelee, Katz, and Lawton (1991), institutionalized elderly with depression, mild depression, and no depression were compared on prevalence for pain complaints. When disability and health factors were controlled, this elderly sample showed no relationship between age and pain intensity or number of localized complaints; however, the authors did find gender differences, with women reporting more intense pain and more pain locations.

This finding has important implications. Because of gender differences in longevity, women represent over 75% of the elderly population sometime after age 75. The question then becomes whether there is a link between gender, psychopathology (specifically prevalence of depression), and pain prevalence in the elderly. There are some suggestions of such interactions in the literature. Kaplan, Barell and Lusky (1988) report evidence that women have more reported depression as well as pain complaints than men throughout their lives. Yet conceivably, this phenomena may reflect reporting bias, since there is also evidence that women generally depict themselves as physically and psychologically less healthy than men. Thus, in any discussion on depression and pain, it is critical to note that pain, gender, and old age interact in a complex manner. According to the National Institute of Mental Health in the United States, mood disorders are less common in the elderly than in younger (middle-aged) individuals, but depression is the reason for admission for nearly half the elderly admitted to psychiatric care (Reiger et al., 1988).

ANXIETY AND CHRONIC PAIN IN THE ELDERLY

Anxiety is another major psychiatric condition associated with chronic pain in the elderly. According to Turnbull (1989), anxiety in the elderly is highly correlated with the experience of chronic pain, chronic ill health, isolation, and the prospect of death following from pain or declining health. Life change issues, such as change in health status, death of friends and intimates, and pain, all commonly experienced by the elderly, may be another contributory factor in the genesis of anxiety.

The most common types of anxiety disorders in the elderly are phobias, anxiety states, and adjustment disorders (Jenike, 1996; Kuch, Cox, Evans, Watson, & Bubela, 1993). The prevalence of anxiety disorders in the elderly especially associated with chronic pain requires that physicians be aware of how these disorders may be manifested in elderly patients. For example, chest pain and palpitation are strongly associated with panic and general anxiety, but headache and chronic pain are more strongly associated with depression (Mayou, 1993). Another finding regarding anxiety is that level of disability or dysfunction associated with chronic pain often stabilizes after 6 months, but the level of anxiety and psychological disturbance typically continues to increase with time (Abbott et al., 1992).

A feature of chronic pain more common in the elderly than in comparable younger age groups is high levels of anxiety related to concerns surrounding death and dying. In one study, data indicated three major categories of fears in the elderly: (1) physical pain and suffering, (2) risk to personal safety, and (3) threat to self-esteem and the uncertainty of life beyond death (Fry, 1990). Elderly persons' memories associated with chronic pain become selective and result in recurrent anxiety surrounding death and suffering. It is also likely that suicide fantasies may not only be associated with clinical depression, but also may be a psychological coping mechanism to give the elderly the feeling of control over the anxiety in situations of illness and pain.

Anxiety, depression, and somatization surrounding chronic pain complaints can take many forms in the elderly. One symptom of psychological distress that appears to be almost universal for elderly chronic pain sufferers is sleep difficulty. In one investigation of night sleep symptoms and their relation to psychological, social, and somatic variables in an elderly population of 162 men and 291 women (aged 75 years and older), it was found that (1) age per se was not a risk factor for a poor night's sleep quality; (2) women reported worse sleep quality (possibly due to the frequent coexistence of depression, anxiety, somatization, disability, and loneliness); and (3) education level was a moderating variable for expectations about sleep quality in the elderly. Additionally, higher levels of somatization and anxiety were independently associated with worse quality of sleep, but depression was not (Frisoni, de Leo, Rozzini, & Bernardini et al., 1993).

ROLE OF MEMORY IMPAIRMENT AS A FACTOR IN CHRONIC PAIN

There are many dimensions of cognitive functioning that can affect the experience of chronic pain in the elderly. A central feature of cognitive functioning is memory. Age-related memory deficit, whether related to or in the absence of cognitive impairment, is an important consideration in understanding chronic pain in the elderly. Long-term memory can be divided into semantic memory, which comprises a person's general knowledge about the world, and episodic memory, which has to do with personally experienced events (Tulving, 1972). Semantic memory performance has been found to be relatively stable across age (Salthouse, 1982). However, the elderly often have been found to have more problems with episodic memory tasks than their younger counterparts (Craik, 1971; Kausler & Wiley, 1991; Light, 1991). Pain memories are typically viewed as episodic in nature. Thus, age-related declines in this aspect of memory could significantly influence the perception of current chronic pain experiences.

Given that memory for past pain experiences is important in forming the basis for an individual's current attitudes, beliefs, and expectations about pain, the question then becomes how common and extensive is memory impairment in the elderly population. In a large North American survey (N = 14,783), approximately 15% of those surveyed over the age of 55 complained of frequent memory problems, while 25% reported none. In this sample, 23% of the oldest-old (age 85+) reported having frequent memory difficulties (Cutler & Grams, 1988).

Morley (1993) found that when memories for everyday events were recalled, vivid memories of painful events were most easily retrieved. When he compared nonpain events and pain events, he found that pain events were characteristically described as more surprising and unexpected and were associated with negative emotional change after the event occurred. Morley also suggested that, because pain events are usually infrequent, they are more memorable. Similar results were found in a study by Rubin and Kozin (1984) on vivid memories. Morley (1993) speculated on several hypotheses as to why understanding memory for pain is crucial. First, psychological accounts of pain phenomena invoke memory for pain as an important component in (1) determining cognitive processing of painful stimuli, (2) shaping the behavioral response to acute pain, and (3) contributing to the establishment of chronic pan behavior. Second, patients are often asked to make judgments about their pain, which implies the use of memory when asked to compare their current pain with past pain experience. Research exploring patients' worst pain memory has found that, with the exception of traumatic pain incidents such as childbirth, individuals of all ages tend to report their most recent pain experience as their most painful experience (Roy, Thomas, & Makarenko, 1990).

COGNITIVE IMPAIRMENT AND PAIN IN THE INSTITUTIONALIZED ELDERLY

The elderly, particularly those in chronic care facilities, have high levels of chronic pain compared to the general population (Ferrini et al., 1993). Roy and Thomas (1986) found that 83% of elderly residents in a nursing home reported pain. This level of pain was further supported by Ferrell, Ferrell, and Osterweil (1990), who reported a 71% prevalence rate of pain in nursing home residents. A continuum of reliability for reported pain in elderly nursing residents clearly exists. On the one end are the cognitively intact, communicative elderly. On the other end are the noncommunicative, cognitively impaired elderly individuals whose pain is detected through inference by caregivers (Sengstaken & King, 1993). Given this situation, the reliability of self-reported pain in elderly patients and nursing home residents can be viewed as being possibly distorted by the level of cognitive impairment. Linton and Melin (1982) found that chronic pain patients after 3–11 weeks of treatment overestimated their pretreatment pain levels. Patients with acute head pain had better memory for their pain, showing slight underestimation (Hunter, Phillips, & Rachman, 1979). Linton and Melin postulated that acute pain such as that in Hunter's study was easier to remember than chronic pain because acute pain was a discrete event that occurred in a specific situation, whereas chronic pain was relatively constant over time and lacked specificity.

Another factor that may account for the difference in memory for acute and chronic pain is the effect of present pain on the memory of pain past. When the level of pain is high at recall, patients tend to underestimate their past pain. When it is low, they overestimate their past pain (Eich, Reeves, Jaeger, & Graft-Radford, 1985). This may have been the case in Linton and Melin's study, because their patients perceived little improvement in their condition, and were thus experiencing high pain at recall. Bryant (1993) further postulated that it was the changes in pain and affect that distorted pain memory. In his study, chronic pain patients who experienced increases in pain and/or depression overestimated their initial pain or depression.

The cognitively impaired have also been found to report less pain than their cognitively intact counterparts (Sengstaken & King,

1993; Parmelee, Smith, & Katz, 1993). The population who experience communicative and cognitive difficulties along with pain may be larger than one might anticipate, especially in an institutionalized setting. Bland, Newman, and Horn (as cited in Health and Welfare Canada, 1991) estimated (conservatively) that 40% of all institutionalized elderly have some sort of dementia. This figure has varied in different studies and has been reported to be as high as one-half or three-quarters of the individuals in the nursing home populations (Hoekstra, Ronbaar, & Laporte, 1996). When this figure is combined with the fact that three-quarters of institutionalized elderly are in pain, a very large number of elderly persons are seemingly influenced by their cognitive status in their pain report.

Memory impairment is considered one of the definitive features of dementia in the elderly, with Alzheimer's disease being the most common classification for this group of elderly as reported in the DSM-IV. Memory loss in the older Alzheimer's patient can be characterized by decrements in all three levels of memory: sensory register, short-term, and long-term memory (Edwards, 1994). Long-term memory can be further divided into semantic and episodic memory, both of which are adversely affected by the presence of dementia. However, an emphasis has been placed on the deterioration of the episodic memory when a clinical diagnosis is being made (Schultz, Schmitt, Logue, & Rubin, as cited in Edwards, 1994). Pain memories are labeled as episodic; therefore, it would be expected that the presence of memory impairment would significantly hamper the accuracy of retrospective pain reports, which in turn impacts the diagnosis of chronic pain versus a current somatic diagnosis.

Hasher and Zacks (1988) have developed a model for encoding memory that differentiates between aging-related memory decline and dementia. Differences on a picturebook task using measures of free recall, recognition accuracy, and memory for location and frequency were found between elderly adult patients on each measure. A discriminate function correctly classified the groups with 93.3% accuracy. Subsequent discriminate analysis found that patients could be correctly classified into diagnostic subgroups (i.e., dementia of the Alzheimer's type, multi-infarct dementia, and Korsakoff's disease) with 80.8% accuracy (Rohling, Ellis, & Scogin, 1991).

ROLE OF DEMENTIA IN CHRONIC PAIN IN THE ELDERLY

Current estimates for the United States project that between 2 and 5 million Americans are currently suffering from some form of dementia (Office of Technology Assessment, cited in Marzinski, 1991). The demographic increase in the older segment of the population is expected to increase the number of dementia cases by 60% by the year 2000 (Marzinski, 1991). In Canada, the number of dementia cases is expected to have doubled in two decades by the year 2006 in the majority of Canadian provinces (Health and Welfare Canada, 1991). The prevalence of dementia, its possible impact on accurate pain diagnosis in the elderly, and its subsequent consequences are clearly a gerontological concern.

Dementia as defined by the American Psychiatric Association (cited in Linderborn, 1988) is an irreversible mental state characterized by a decrease in intellectual function, personality change, impaired judgment, and often a change in affect (Folstein, Anthony, Parhad, Duffy, & Gruenberg, 1985). The most obvious and serious impact dementia has on chronic pain in the elderly is their ability to relay subjective pain information accurately; otherwise, there is the possibility that chronic pain may be ignored, undertreated, or assumed to be nonexistent (Parmelee et al., 1993; Sengstaken & King, 1993). Chronic pain among nonverbal elderly or severely cognitively impaired individuals usually is expressed in the form of stereotypical pain behaviors, such as moaning, whimpering, withdrawal, restlessness, guarding, and protective postures (Herr & Mobily, 1991). Other stereotyped pain behaviors include recognizing changes in routine, gait, facial expression, posture changes, diaphoresis, and pupillary changes (Marzinski, 1991). Even those with severe cognitive dysfunctions are likely to exhibit stereotypical pain behavior (Hurley, Volicer, Hanrahan, Hourda, & Volier, 1992). Regardless of the severity of pain, it has been noted that nurses chart less than 50% of what elderly patients describe (Marzinski, 1991). This could be attributed to cultural views of pain, ageism (that pain is an inherent and expected part of aging), or simply that nurses do not believe patients with perceived or real cognitive impairment.

The most prevalent form of dementia is Alzheimer's disease. This neurological disease is diagnosed in 50% of all cases of senile dementia, which is the progressive deterioration of cognitive abilities to dysfunctional levels in the social and occupational spheres. In a large survey in the United States conducted by the National Institute of Mental Health, it was found that only a small proportion of persons under age 60 are diagnosed with dementia, while approximately 20% of persons 80 years old and older were diagnosed with dementia (LaRue, Dessonville, & Jarvik, 1985).

In a large sample study, the association between self-reported pain and cognitive impairment among 758 frail elderly institution residents (mean age 83.3 years) was investigated (Parmelle et al., 1993). The subjects' self-reports included pain intensity, number of localized pain complaints, cognitive status, and disability in performance of activities of daily living. Pain intensity and number of localized pain complaints bore small but significant negative relationships to cognitive impairment. Pain was positively associated with physician-rated ill health and functional disability. There were no differences between pain reports of cognitively impaired versus intact elderly in either the presence or absence of a likely physical cause. The data also provided no evidence for the masking of pain complaints by cognitive impairment. Although the cognitively impaired elderly tended to slightly underreport experienced pain, their self-reports were generally no less valid than those of cognitively intact individuals (Parmelee et al., 1993).

CONCLUSIONS

The literature indicates relatively high prevalence rates of chronic pain in the elderly, which is a growing part of the general population. Yet, the research focusing on pain experiences of this population is still only a minimal proportion of the overall pain research. Less than 1% of the pain literature in any given year is devoted to pain research with the elderly (Jacox, Carr, & Payne, 1994).

The causes and expressions of mental disorders that are most common in their affect on chronic pain are usually assumed to be uniform across all adults age groups even though there is no strong empirical basis for this "uniformity" assumption. When looking at all combined psychiatric disorders in the DSM-III-R, comparisons for different age groups found that persons over 65 had the lowest prevalence rates. Specifically, the prevalence of Somatization, Hypochondriasis, and Delusional Disorder Somatic Type in persons over 65 is a minimal percent of this population. This is consistent with most research that has not found a direct relationship between psychopathology and the physiological processes of aging. The one obvious exception to this finding is the high association between pain, depressed affect, and age (Roy et al., 1984; Parmelee et al., 1989; Sullivan et al., 1991; Hodgkiss, 1997). The most commonly given explanation for this age and pain relationship involves the cognitive–behavioral mediation model of depression in chronic pain where cognitive appraisal variables are hypothesized to mediate the pain–depression relationship. Consistent with this cognitive–behavioral model, younger patients typically demonstrate a low and nonsignificant correlation between pain severity and depression. Conversely, a strong direct association is common in the older patients between pain severity and depression (Turk et al., 1995).

There are other conditions of pathology both psychological and physical that impact the reporting and experience of chronic pain in the elderly residing in the community and in institutional settings. In addition to depression, anxiety and somatic expression of emotional distress psychologically influence the reporting of chronic pain in the elderly. Specifically, there are fears and anxieties of dying associated with chronic pain among the elderly in greater proportion than in other age cohorts. This relationship would appear bidirectional in that fear of dying may exaggerate reported pain as well.

Another area investigated in the pain literature is cognitive functioning in the elderly and its impact on the pain prevalence in this group. One reason for the interest in this area is because associations between age, pain perception, memory, and dementia have been established. However, there is a general tendency for the elderly as an age cohort to report less pain than younger age cohorts. What mechanisms (psychological or physiological) that may be responsible for this phenomena are still highly speculative. Although aging is typically associated with higher pain tolerances, this phenomenon in community samples of the elderly may be even further exacerbated in institutionalized elderly by higher incidences of dementia and memory impairment that may mask chronic pain reporting.

In summary, chronic pain is present in the elderly but not typically associated with psychological etiology or prevalence. Rather, psychological factors and cognitive impairment appear more related to coping with chronic pain than as a primary determinate of pain prevalence in the elderly. Gibson et al. (1994) reviewed the physiological, pathological, and psychological reasons for pain reporting in older persons. Their conclusion was that altered physiology of pain mechanisms combined with psychological attitudes, such as stoicism and reluctance to confirm the presence of pain, give rise to higher pain thresholds in the elderly. However, the elderly describe the same severity and quality of pain experience and psychological disturbance associated with chronic pain as do younger persons. As an example of this phenomena, one study that compared physical and psychosocial characteristics of 60 elderly chronic pain patients (aged 60 years and older) and 60 younger patients (aged 35 years and younger) found that although older patients had more frequent abnormal physical findings, there were no significant differences on measures of self-reported activity, pain severity, life interference, or emotional or worry reactions in response to pain. Both age groups had comparable scores on measures of social support and perceptions of how others react to their pain (Sorkin et al., 1990).

Emotional and behavioral disturbances provoked by chronic pain in the elderly are significant and should not be dismissed as "normal aging phenomena" or treated any less aggressively by professionals. The presence of persistent or recurrent clinical pain has a significant impact on the psychological, social, and physical functioning of older adults. Prohaska et al. (1985) found that the elderly reported feeling more vulnerable to illness, that illness is more serious in its possible consequences for them, and that pain is the primary trigger for these concerns. Symptoms associated with illness in general by the elderly were pain, tiredness, lack of energy, weakness, and sleeplessness.

CHAPTER 10

Social and Family Issues and the Elderly Chronic Pain Patient

In this chapter, we shall examine some of the more critical life events commonly faced by the elderly and the role of social support. In addition, family problems and conflicts will be scrutinized. It must be emphasized that the actual literature on these topics related to the elderly chronic pain patient is somewhat sparse. Much of the material presented here is drawn from the general literature on the elderly with health problems. The case illustrations will confirm that many problems are commonly shared by the elderly by virtue of their life stage, and the problems are further complicated by virtue of their health problems.

CASE ILLUSTRATION

This case encompasses many of the critical problems in the areas of life events, social support, and family issues not uncommon in the elderly with chronic pain or illness. This is the story of Mrs. A, aged 67, who was referred to this author following a rather dramatic deterioration of her head and back pain. Neurological and orthopedic investigations were negative. She had a lifelong history of headaches, which had not presented a serious challenge to her well-being. Her back pain also had a 25-year history. Despite her prolonged history of pain, she had led a full life. She had hardly ever sought medical help with her pain. However, on this occasion, she consulted her family physician who placed her on narcotic and nonnarcotic analgesics as well as antidepressant medication. Mrs. A failed to respond, and was subsequently referred to the pain clinic.

Mrs. A along with her husband were seen for routine psychosocial investigation. They had a traditional marriage in that Mr. A was the main breadwinner and Mrs. A was a lifelong homemaker. Both were successful in their pursuits. Mr. A was a successful businessman and for much of his working life had traveled throughout the world, spending little time at home. Mrs. A raised five children "almost singlehanded," she claimed. She described her husband as somewhat peripheral to the family system, though in recent years he had grown closer to the children. He angrily rejected her description of his peripheral role. He had a very responsible position which kept him away from his family, but he tried to spend as much time as he could with the family. He portrayed his wife as a perfectionist, overbearing, and always expecting too much from him. Despite these chronic conflicts, all five children were pursuing successful careers in various professions. They acknowledged that since their father's retirement, their relationship had deteriorated rather sharply. This was the first indication of a major, though not unexpected, life event they had recently experienced.

Since his retirement, her husband had intruded into her daily life in a wholly unacceptable way. He showed very little regard for her daily routine, and sat reading the newspaper in the kitchen for hours on end. He refused to shave unless he had to, and worst of all wore the same underclothes for 2 or 3 days in a row. Then there was a dramatic development. He claimed serious hearing loss. Mrs. A would be blasting away at him about this and that, and he would sit without as much as moving a muscle. This drove Mrs. A to distraction. He was examined by the family physician who could not find any hearing abnormality. Her headaches took a turn for the worse, which seriously affected her day-to-day life. On some days she could not even get out of bed. On these occasions, Mr. A would be a changed man, being overly solicitous and "unendingly" fussing over his wife. As soon as her headaches improved, he would return to his "obnoxious self."

Conceptually, all three issues relevant to this chapter were evident in this case. The major life event for Mr. and Mrs. A was indeed Mr. A's retirement. This is an event that is not necessarily undesirable and most certainly is predictable. In that sense this event did not have to be perceived as negative. Mr. A's attitude toward retirement was mixed. He welcomed the absence of endless travel, which left him with ample time to "please himself." He missed his lifelong friends in the business world, but he had joined a golf club to compensate for that. Mrs. A's response was almost entirely negative. This only worsened with each passing day. She saw him as lazy, uncooperative, and generally a nuisance. The point here is that while much of the literature on life events is concerned with the individual experiencing the event(s), intimates are also affected by these events. In this particular instance, Mr. A's retirement had a far worse effect on his wife.

In terms of social support, some intriguing changes occurred. Mrs. A was reluctant to invite her friends home to save herself the "embarrassment" of exposing her unkempt husband, and her worsening pain prevented her from remaining engaged in the community. Mr. A, as stated, missed his friends from work, but this did not leave a very serious gap in his life. He was busy planning for his retired existence. However, as the literature will testify, retirement is often a mixed blessing. It should be noted that this couple was financially well-off and retirement did not create any hardship.

In terms of family relationship, the role of retirement and Mrs. A's pain problems were quite revealing. From the view of interpersonal relationships, the "message" value or the metaphorical aspect of Mrs. A's pain is instructive. At its simplest, the pain was a powerful message for expressing dissatisfaction with her life situation precipitated by her husband's retirement. At a more complex level, pain served the purpose of correcting what family theorists have described as "hierarchical incongruity." This concept is predicated on the assumption that while a symptomatic partner in a marriage assumes a dependent position, symptoms also have the capacity to empower that person, which in turn rectifies the power imbalance in marriage (Madanes, 1981).

In short, pain enables the person in the position below to gain the upper hand. Mr. A, having lost his power and authority in the business world, by becoming a "slob," he virtually destroyed Mrs. A's assumptive world and the control she had exercised over this world all her married life. His desire to basically ignore her world was challenged only when Mrs. A's pain reached a high level of disability. In that situation, Mrs. A regained some of her authority by forcing him into an unfamiliar nurturing role and on these occasions Mrs. A was listened to literally and figuratively. Mrs. A regained some of her power by becoming symptomatic. Here it must be emphasized that the mechanism involved in Mrs. A's increasing pain is far from simple. It is almost always unconscious, and frequently psychophysiological processes, such as increased stress contributing to more muscle tension and more pain, may be involved.

Rarely, a phenomenon of this kind is a sign of malingering. The most important observation from an interpersonal view related to this case is that age does not preclude serious challenges to marital stability, and assessment and treatment of these interpersonal issues are paramount. Another factor is worthy of attention. Pain in the absence of discernible organic reason tends to be explained in intrapsychic or psychodynamic terms. For example, a persuasive case can be made that Mrs. A's pain symptoms were signs of hysterical or conversion reaction or somatoform disorder. For our purpose, the explanation we sought was interpersonal. The latter is a rather neglected conceptual or explanatory model to describe psychogenic pain. Another point is that regardless of the etiology of pain, the interpersonal elements still play a significant role. Pain or illness in one member can potentially and often does have far-reaching consequences for all intimates. This particular aspect is generally ignored by intrapsychic models.

In the remainder of this chapter, we shall review, albeit with a broad brush, the relevant literature on life events, focusing on retirement, social support, and family issues in the elderly; we will seek empirical validity for some of our observations related to the case of Mr. and Mrs. A.

LIFE EVENTS

In reviewing the life transition and life events literature, we must acknowledge that the actual transition that involved our couple only affected Mrs. A. Nevertheless, to state the obvious, a single event can generate a series of related events. In this case, however, the event did not in itself create new events, but had a profound impact on the marriage and health of the spouse. A great deal of the literature on old age and life events seems to be centered on life events and psychological health in general, and life events and depression in particular. Unlike the younger chronic pain population, where a body of research connecting life event with pain problems exists, such literature is rather scarce with the elderly. Life event issues in relation to old age have been examined from a variety of perspectives: life events and anxiety (Wheatley, 1988), neurosis (Rangaswami, 1983), health perceptions (Duckitt, 1983), psychological well-being (Frischer, Ford, & Taylor, 1991), depression (Baldwin, 1991), and so on. The life events literature is rather silent on the consequences of life event on the intimates.

In recent years a plethora of studies have been reported on many aspects of life events and their association with pain disorders. This body of literature is confined mostly, though not exclusively, to middle-aged chronic pain patients. The impact of life events has been investigated with pain conditions as varied as headaches (deBenditis, Lorenzetti, & Pieri, 1990; deBendittis & Lorenzetti, 1992), chronic low back pain (Atkinson et al., 1988; Smith et al., 1985), irritable bowel syndrome (Fowlie, Eastwood, & Ford, 1992), facial pain (Lennon et al., 1990; Zaruta et al., 1995), and abdominal pain (Jenkins, 1991; Johnson & Theorell, 1991), and this is only a partial list. Findings have been mixed in the sense that while some studies have shown a strong association between negative life events and onset of illness or worsening of an existing illness, other studies simply have failed to find such a relationship. Several studies challenged the notion that life events played any significant role in the etiology of pain disorders (Feuerstein et al., 1985; Pilowsky & Bassett, 1982; Jensen, 1988; Marback et al., 1988; Stockton, Weinman, & McCall, 1985). A few studies found an association between life events and higher level of distress, but no clear association emerged between life events and pain (Klages, 1991; Zaruta et al., 1995). In short, while there is mounting evidence of an intricate relationship between onset of pain and recent negative life events, the idea of a linear relationship between life events and chronic pain disorders remains somewhat equivocal, thus demonstrating the complex nature of this association.

Nevertheless, retirement as an event has come under some scrutiny. Matthew and Brown (1987) investigated the experience of retirement in a group of 176 men and 124 women in the age range of 60 to 72 years. One of the central findings of this study was that retirement was far less problematic than previous research had indicated. Men and women reacted somewhat differentially to this event, and pre-retirement planning had an effect on the reaction and adaptation to retirement. In a study of retirement as a life event, Szinovacz and Washo (1992) found that in a group of 441 women and 370 men aged between 50 and 85 years, women reported more life events prior to retirement and they were also more adversely affected postretirement than men. Regardless of gender, however, subjects with more education and better health adapted more easily to retirement than others.

There are several papers addressing the question of pain and retirement. Herr and Mobily (1991) discussed the complexities of pain assessment in the elderly and how this process is complicated by psychosocial factors such as retirement. It should be noted that this was not an empirically based paper. In a Finnish study, Harkappa (1992) investigated the association between chronic low back pain and retirement, and in a follow-up study found that early retirement was associated with free-floating anxiety, internal locus of control, and belief in control by others, among other factors.

Another body of relevant literature examined the relationship between retirement and depression. Benefits of retirement planning on mental health (Midanik, Soghikian, Ransom, & Tekawa, 1995), effects of gender and occupational level on the psychological consequences of retirement (de Grace, Joshi, & Pelletier, 1994), depression following retirement (Muller-Spahn & Hock, 1994), and the broader psychosocial consequences of retirement (Luscher, 1993) may be considered only a partial list of recent publications on this topic. One fact is inescapable. Studies designed to study the positive aspects of retirement are difficult to find.

One study that has some relevance to our case examined the relationship between household labor inequality and retirement-aged wives' marital and personal happiness (Pina & Bengston, 1995). Results based on a survey of 144 women aged 54 to 74 years found that household labor inequality was inversely related to positive interaction, closeness, and affirmation of the wife. Wives who were satisfied with their husbands' support experienced less negative aspects of marital quality and reported less depression (Pina & Bengston, 1995). In the case of Mrs. A, her husband, at least in her judgment, was always peripheral to the family by virtue of his prolonged absence from home due to business. His retirement resulted in a major reorganization in their family relationship. Having lost his main role as the breadwinner of the family and never having any other significant role, he was viewed more as an intruder by Mrs. A. The fact that he was never particularly supportive of her was now compounded by his perceived unreasonable conduct. Those circumstances presumably contributed to the development of her symptoms.

Retirement is unquestionably a momentous event in a person's life. As Floyd and associates (1992) note that unlike childhood developmental milestones, which are relatively invariant, the principle of contextualism proposes that individual experiences surrounding adult transitions determine the meaning and impact of the transitions for different persons. Thus, although transitions such as retirement are normative, and the event itself is usually predictable and planned, the contexts for different individuals create differences in how this transition comes about, the meaning of the event, the short-term adjustments required, and the long-term impact of the event on the individual's life.

So much of personal worth is tied up with work that giving it up or forced retirement is an event of considerable emotional significance. As noted, much of the literature is concerned with negative outcome of retirement. Literature dealing with the complex nature of retirement is emerging. Floyd et al. (1992) developed a measure of retirement as a life transition. In the course of the investigation, they interviewed a substantial number of men and women who had recently retired. As a result of their investigation, they identified six domains: preretirement work functioning, adjustment, and change; reasons for retirement; sources of support in retirement; and leisure and physical activities. These variables provide a comprehensive view of retirees' perception of the impact of retirement as well as predict level of adjustment to retirement.

In our case, Mr. A, the retiree, was less affected by his retirement than was his wife. The impact of retirement on the spouse remains an uncharted territory. Nevertheless, it is reasonable to assume, as in the case of Mrs. A, that retirement can have far-reaching consequences for a marriage for the simple reason that rules by which couples have lived are somewhat suddenly changed. In the section that follows, we shall explore the family issues confronted by the elderly in general and chronic pain sufferers in particular.

FAMILY ISSUES

Over the past 20 years, there has been an explosion of publications on the topic of chronic pain and family (see Chapter 7). Unfortunately, almost all that literature is confined to the middle-aged pain clinic populations. Family problems of the elderly chronic pain sufferer remain, by and large, unexplored.

Family issues confronted by the elderly chronic pain patients are the same and yet very different than their younger counterparts. Life stage is a major determinant of the family issues. Interpersonal conflicts do not seem to diminish with age (Hughston, Christopherson, & Bonjean, 1989). Retirement, widowhood, availability of friends, and existence of a social network; contact with and support from children; health of the spouse; and financial stability are some of the critical family issues for the elderly. Family functioning, for a vast majority of the elderly, translates into couple functioning. It is worth recalling that almost all studies related to family problems of the chronic pain population, which is primarily drawn from pain clinics, found wide-ranging difficulties. Unfortunately, there is a dearth of such studies with the elderly chronic pain population, and much of what is discussed here is from extrapolation of related literature.

Family relationships among the elderly, as is evident even from our case illustration, can assume great complexity. Unfortunately, study of families of the elderly from a systemic view are very rare. Many reports are to be found in the literature on elderly families covering a very broad range of problematic areas. A few of those reports are briefly discussed. Field, Minkler, Falk, and Leino (1993), in a longitudinal study involving 62 subjects aged 74 to 93 years, found that subjects in better health had greater amounts of contact with family than did those in poorer health. And an Indian study involving 720 retired men found that life satisfaction was derived from activities associated with their occupation, hobbies, friends, and voluntary organizations (Mishra, 1992). Religious and household activities and interaction with family members and neighbors had no such impact on life satisfaction.

These two studies are presented to show that the centrality of the family in the well-being of the elderly, especially among the healthy, is not an incontrovertible truth. Nevertheless, there is evidence that support of the family member is often crucial for the well-being of the elderly. Shanas (1979) reported that among the housebound non-institutionalized elderly, the spouse was often the only source of support. In a later study, she found that as people were living longer, the burden of caregiving was being assumed to an increasing degree by children and grandchildren (Shanas, 1984). Greene (1989) commented on the phenomenon of the rising number of multigenerational families, and three- and four-generation families were no longer uncommon. Sudden health problems in the older members created a bewildering effect on the entire family system. Children and grandchildren often found themselves involved in complex and highly stressful family situations.

Another point is that elderly persons for the most part live alone or with spouses. In order to comprehend the nature and extent of marital and family conflict, it is necessary to examine the family and couples therapy literature pertaining to this population. One major problem with this body of literature is that much of it is nonempirical. Two themes emerge: (1) Marital and family problems do not necessarily diminish with age, and (2) illness and disability in a spouse are not uncommon causes for exacerbation of marital conflict. Another obvious observation is that if a couple has lived in a state of conflict throughout their marriage, attaining senior status does nothing to alter the relationship.

To return to the first theme—that marital difficulties do not decrease in old age—Ruskin (1985) reported on 67 patients over the age of 60 who were referred to the gerontopsychiatric service of a teaching hospital. Twenty-five percent were faced with family problems and family therapy was the treatment of choice. In another study, 20 hypochondriacal patients over the age of 60 were grouped into primary and secondary hypochondriasis. Four patients were in the former group and benefitted little from treatment. In the latter group, family therapy along with other interventions were offered. The point to note is that family problems were endemic in this selected group of patients (Goldstein & Birnbaum, 1976).

A recent report by Meunier (1994) suggests that the most common cause for marital therapy for elderly couples is illness of a spouse. Another common reason is one member grows while the other remains entrenched. The conclusion to be drawn is that any major change in the pattern of living, which has evolved over a very long period of time, puts marriage under strain. In a study of 900 respondents between the ages of 65 and 94, married women had the poorest health and were found to be most vulnerable to stress (Preston & Dellasega, 1990). Subjects were divided into the following categories: Those with (1) poor health and low stress; (2) poor health and high stress; (3) good health and low stress; and (4) good health and high stress. For our purposes, the point is that the burden of coping with a sick partner often falls on the wives. This is especially evident in the caregiving literature, which falls outside the scope of this chapter.

Beckham and Giordano (1986) observed the problems associated with offering marital therapy to couples when one partner is impaired by disease or disability. They found that preexisting marital difficulties, reluctance to admit difficulty in coping, compounded by low income were major barriers to marital therapy. This paper helps explain, at least in part, the vulnerability of the caregiver to stress due to failure to accept help.

Self-referral for marital conflict among the aged remains problematic (Mosher, 1993). Only 11% in a group of 298 elderly clients of a community mental center were self-referred. Professional assessment of these cases revealed that a vast majority of community residents either had depression and/or family conflicts. In addition, the task of diagnosing family conflict was primarily carried out by social workers, as few referrals for marital problems were made by physicians (Mosher, 1993). A Russian study involving 120 psychiatrically impaired subjects between the ages of 47 and 73 years found that all subjects had family conflicts (Danilov & Selivra, 1990).

One study investigated the family functioning of nine patients aged 65 and over attending a pain clinic and their spouses (R. Roy, unpublished data). One year was needed to obtain this small sample of elderly persons at the pain clinic. The Family Adaptability and Cohesion Evaluation Scale (FACES III) was used to assess family function. On the Family Adaptability Scale, which measures a family's capacity to adapt to altered life situations brought on by illness and other factors, only one couple was found to be functioning in the effective or "flexible" range. Three couples showed almost total failure to adapt and the rest showed varying levels of difficulty in adapting to altered situations. Couples revealed a remarkable degree of agreement on their difficulty to adapt to change.

On Family Cohesion, which purports to measure emotional bonding between family members, three couples were connected, four were disengaged, one enmeshed, and one presented a mixed picture of being disengaged and separated. Two thirds of this group reported some level of difficulty in the domain of emotional support. Again, the couples reported a very high level of agreement on Family Cohesion. A word of caution is necessary. This was only a pilot study. The hope was to mount a controlled study at a later date. That proved impossible, as the annual rate of inception of elderly patients at the pain clinic remained extremely low.

However, there are some contrary data. Bishop, Epstein, Keitner, Miller, and Srinivasan (1986) investigated family functioning of victims of stroke in elderly subjects, mean age 65 years, 1 year after the stroke. They found that family function as measured by Family Assessment Devise (FAD) was mainly unaffected by stroke. The subjects were carefully selected on the basis of their capacity to attend an outpatient rehabilitation program. This may suggest that this group of patients was not seriously damaged by the stroke.

The literature on marital and family therapy with the elderly is also revealing in terms of the sheer variety of interpersonal problems and the innovations in adapting these therapies to the elderly. However, outcome studies for family and marital therapies are nonexistent with this population. The volume of clinical literature on the application of family therapy with the elderly is substantial. Only a brief summary of that literature is discussed. In the recent past, conjoint therapy (LaWall, 1981), community intervention (Garrison & Howe, 1976), group treatment for well spouses (Beaulieu & Karpinsky, 1981), crisis intervention with elderly couples (Getzel, 1982), an ecological approach dealing with the transitional tasks (Lee, 1989), and many more approaches have come under the scrutiny of family therapists in their work with the elderly.

In more recent times, family therapy for elderly patients with dementia (Goldstein, 1990; Huckle, 1994), those at risk for psychiatric disorders in a general practice in the United Kingdom (Carpenter, 1994), to resolve conflicts with family members (Virtanen, 1993), for depression (Molinari, 1991; Woods, 1993), to deal with alcoholism (Amodeo, 1990), and other related topics have been reported. It should be noted that outcome of family therapy with the elderly medically ill, as with all medically ill irrespective of age, remains a neglected field (Roy & Frankel, 1995). Clinical applications of this therapy with young and old alike are voluminous (Roy, 1989, 1990, 1995).

Reasons for this oversight are many and complex. The biomedical orientation of medicine in general is certainly a major contributory factor. In relation to the elderly, ageism or age discrimination cannot be ignored. This has been demonstrated with increasing vigor in the literature dealing with the absence of psychological interventions with the elderly chronic pain patients (Sorkin & Turk, 1995). Resistance on the part of the professionals to use family therapy for older adults has also been noted (Gilleard, Lieberman, & Feeler, 1992). They surveyed 15 physicians, 15 nurses, and 10 social workers to discover that "there was a mixture of ignorance about the service (family therapy) in particular and the approach in general, as well as some reservations concerning the potential for change in the families of older adults (p. 415).

Carpenter's (1994) study, based in England, is of some importance as it tried to investigate the patterns of referral of elderly patients deemed to be at some psychiatric risk. Fifty-four referrals over a period of 3 years were investigated. Results showed that 30% of the referrals mentioned marital or family problems. Family issues remained the focus of intervention in 40% of these cases. Only 9% qualified for conjoint sessions as a primary means of therapy. Carpenter buttressed his plea for a family orientation by discussing cases to show the importance of family systems ideas both in understanding and treating them.

A Finnish report strongly recommended incorporation of family assessment into routine gerontopsychiatric interviews (Virtanen,

1993). Interactional problems between family members were found to be common. The goal of family therapy, in this approach, was to help the family accept one's own and the family's life cycle issues rather than concrete changes in the future (Virtanen, 1993).

The final report is another British study in a general practice setting that reviewed 104 referrals for family therapy (Graham, Senior, Dukes, & Lazarus, 1993). Clients showed a high rate of acceptance for this treatment. Several cases were presented to show the beneficial effects of family therapy for all age groups (Graham et al., 1993).

The gap in our knowledge about family issues in the elderly chronic pain population is nothing short of embarrassing. And yet common sense dictates that family issues cannot and indeed do not vaporize in old age. This observation received considerable support in a comprehensive review of research literature (discussed in the next section) on the benefits of family support for elderly chronically ill persons (Kriegsman, Penninx, & van Eijk, 1995). They concluded that active involvement of close family members and discussion of marital difficulties had a positive influence on an elderly patient's mental and physical health. A family-oriented approach in counseling elderly patients with chronic diseases could also have a positive impact on the process of rehabilitation. This very important review paper will be discussed in some detail in the following section. The limited clinical and anecdotal information we have on the elderly chronic pain patient, supported by literature on other groups of elderly persons and their families, clearly calls for more attention to family issues and conflicts.

SOCIAL SUPPORT

Social and interpersonal environments not only exert a profound influence on a person's mental health, but also have considerable significance for physical health (Hinkle, 1961). Even earlier, Hinkle and Wolfe (1957) observed that one's satisfaction with life was in considerable measure dependent on strong and stable family ties. In more recent years this theoretical proposition has obtained much empirical respectability. A plethora of research has purported to show that availability of social support serves a clear function in moderating the effects of a variety of disorders. At a more general level, social support is now generally accepted as a critical area of investigation in the overall social environment of the patient.

Social support in old age has been long recognized as an important variable in the well-being of that population. Several studies showed that social support has a moderating effect on depression in the elderly (Oppegard et al., 1984; Pahkala, 1990; Woo, Ho, Lau, Yuen, et al., 1994). However, the evidence is more complex than suggested. One study found that social support among other factors was more critical in influencing depression in younger adults, while poor physical health exerted far greater influence on depression in the elderly (McNeil & Harsany, 1989). Another study reported that loneliness in a group of elderly was far more a function of physical impairment, a lack of confidantes, low morale, and low life satisfaction. The quality of a confiding relationship proved to be of much greater value than the quantity of social support (Mellor & Edelman, 1988). Another rather contradictory finding was that among the elderly, women, whites, those living alone, and those with low education and greater strain were also likely to receive more social support, although they tended to have smaller sources of support (Arling, 1987). This study is especially important as it shows that a group most in need of social support is also very vulnerable.

Our focus will be on the relationship of social support and its moderating influence on chronic pain. There are only a handful of reports on the influence of social support on chronic pain (Cook & Thomas, 1994; Gaston-Johansson et al., 1990; Goldberg et al., 1993; Helme, Gibson, & Farrell, 1996; Jamison & Virts, 1990; Weickgenant et al., 1993; Weir, Browne, Tunks, & Gafni, 1992). Only two of these papers (Helme et al. and Cook & Thomas) were concerned with the elderly.

Cook and Thomas (1994) investigated the role of social support in a group of 112 community-dwelling elderly persons. Forty-two percent of these individuals reported chronic pain. Although the pain group reported more health problems than the nonpain subjects, there was no difference between the two groups on the mean score on perceived social support. However, the pain group had significantly more hassles in their daily lives. Cook and Thomas hypothesized that among other variables, the pain group had less effective social support, which enhanced their vulnerability to pain and heightened level of stress.

Helme et al. (1996) explored the influence of social support on the chronic pain experience in an elderly population in Australia. The sample consisted of 214 consecutive patients (mean age 73.7 years) attending a geriatric pain management clinic. Their findings were complex and contradictory. They found that increased utilization of social and support services such as home help, meals on wheels, and so on, was associated with increased anxiety, depression, and functional impairment. Conversely, social support while having a moderating effect on depression through a greater sense of control, was also associated with greater pain. Social support was seen as more desirable, as it moderated the negative effects of chronic pain, but social services were seen as somewhat counterproductive for chronic pain. They did not offer any explanation for this intriguing finding. Of note was that community services and social support accounted for only 5% of the variance, thus revealing their very limited effect.

To further appreciate the complexity surrounding the question of the value of social support, Taal, Rasker, Seydel, and Wiegman (1993), in a group of 86 patients with rheumatoid arthritis (mean age 60 years), found that while emotional social support did not influence self-efficacy, "instrumental" support was positively related to health status. This finding is somewhat contradictory to Helme's study reported in the previous paragraph.

In general terms, these reports taken together support the proposition that social support exerts a positive influence in moderating the ill effects of chronic pain. This, however, is not a universal fact. Several studies question the unequivocal benefit of social support, again in studies with younger chronic pain populations. Two studies have failed to find any direct beneficial or buffering of chronic pain conditions by social support (Bradley et al., 1992; Faucett & Levine, 1991). These studies involved rather divergent pain populations.

There is another body of literature that reveals rather mixed results. We shall summarize the key findings of a major review of the research literature on family support and chronic illness (Kriegsman et al., 1995). The part of the review that has direct relevance for this chapter is the role of family support for patients suffering from rheumatoid arthritis and osteoarthritis. Findings are mixed at best. One study confirmed the hypothesis that social support could exert a buffering effect (Weinberger, Tierney, Boober, & Hiner, 1990). Lower levels of physical functioning were associated with lower levels of tangible support as well as support directed at improving self-esteem in a group of patients with osteoarthritis. In another study, Weinberger, Hiner, and Tierney (1987) showed that married osteoarthritic patients had less physical disability compared to single patients. However, in a 15-month follow-up study of patients with physical disability, Fitzpatrick, Newman, Lamb, and Shipley (1988) found no such association. This study received further support in a study of patients with rheumatoid arthritis that failed to establish any relationship between quality of social support and physical functioning (Goodenow, Reisine, & Grady, 1990). The reviewers concluded that the part played by social support in the process of disease development remained unclear. They recognized that the review was confined to only one source of support. Nevertheless, these contradictory findings demand more and better-designed investigations.

SUMMARY

This chapter has considered the broader social context of a chronic pain sufferer. Incorporation of these aspects of a patient's life paint a more complex and yet a more realistic portrait of the patient's predicament. Family issues, life events, and social support are only some of the elements in a patient's environment. Some of the very critical issues such as a patient's financial situation, leisure activities, living conditions, and so on, however, are still excluded from our consideration.

In previous studies, we have examined pain in a healthy group of elderly persons (Roy & Thomas, 1987, 1988). We drew our subjects from a social organization that provided all variety of activities, from swimming and aerobics to cards and chess. Many subjects in this group lived with chronic and at times severe pain. Yet, they were a highly functional group almost totally devoid of depression. We concluded that belonging to a social organization that gave them a sense of belonging, friendships, and meaningful activities enabled this group of elderly people to function at a very high level.

The preoccupation in the scientific literature is, as it must be, to establish either etiologic significance of family factors and life events or the buffering power of social support. In clinical practice, however, these issues are clearly important. If a person has experienced recent negative life events, is faced with serious family conflict, or has little in the way of social support, it is reasonable to assume that these circumstances are more than likely to have a negative influence on the patient's well-being. In short, for the clinician to have an adequate understanding of the patient behind the pain, these issues must be explored. There is the added risk with the elderly that these factors will be overlooked.

CHAPTER 11

Epilogue

In this volume, we undertook the challenge of reporting chronic pain across primarily the adult human lifespan. Infancy, childhood, and for the most part adolescent phases were only minimally touched on. So, in reality, the volume is primarily concerned with chronic pain during adulthood. In this chapter, we will indulge in some personal reflections, focusing on some of our salient observations and considering their clinical importance.

First, chronic pain in one form or another appears to be ubiquitous throughout the entire lifespan. Study after study attests to that fact. Whereas traditionally pain has been seen as a natural accompaniment of old age, many studies now have confirmed the common presence of pain complaints in virtually every age group. In fact, the Nuprin Report (Sternbach, 1986) did a great service by confirming that other than joint pain, which was more common in the elderly, younger people had more pain complaints than the elderly. Our own research with the college student population has shown that pain symptoms are experienced by a vast number of them. The middle years are often seen as the beginning of chronic pain problems. Perhaps this view needs to be modified in light of established and still emerging information about the presence of chronic pain problems in younger age groups.

Life stage issues have a rather complex way of complicating pain experiences. Apart from the fact that certain painful diseases are age-specific, life events as well as family and larger social factors appear to be just as relevant to the pain experience as the life stage of our patients. The experiences of life, from entering early adulthood, which could mean leaving home and the familiar environments like high school, to enter the stressful environs of a university with all that it implies, to the isolation of the sick elderly and the reality of serious life changes, conspire to influence the pain experience in rather unpredictable ways.

We have argued that the literature has somewhat narrowly focused on the etiologic significance of a phenomenon such as life events, and the verdict is yet to be delivered. While that line of investigation is critical, the social and psychological impact of such changes in coping with an ongoing chronic pain problem may be of great clinical import. It is not an uncommon experience for many pain clinicians to have a patient lose her or his job or go through a divorce or experience the death of a parent. Common sense suggests that any of these experiences may influence the pain experience and/or the pain behavior of the patient. Our point is that stresses and strains associated with specific life stage must be recognized in order to properly assess the pain issues. The question is the extent to which clinicians are consciously aware of these issues and have developed ways of addressing them.

The role of the family to help or hinder in the treatment of our patients is another area of much importance. While esoteric debate takes place in the learned journals about the pros and cons of family support, the fact is that there is overwhelming evidence to show that family support can be of monumental value to the patient. As clinicians we try to usurp this support to the benefit of the patient and the family. In spite of the rapid decline in nuclear families in North America, the family as a central source of support continues to be critical when addressing chronic pain.

Again, age-specific family issues in relation to chronic pain are relevant. For an elderly pain patient, who is solely reliant on an aged partner, the issues are fundamentally different than those of a middle-aged patient who has abrogated all parental and spousal roles, thus placing the entire family system under great strain. Both families could be at risk. In relation to the young adult, we found pain to be a common experience for family members. We also noted the complex issues surrounding the sharing of pain sites between parents and children. The implications are not altogether clear. At the level of speculation, modeling may be the operating phenomena. In any event, that pain is a family matter for many young persons deserves greater attention from researchers and clinicians alike.

Family issues have the potential of enormous variation at different life stages. First, it is important to acknowledge that much of the family research is confined to the middle-aged pain clinic population. The weight of the evidence points in the direction of a multitude of problems in these families. Such data are virtually absent for all other age groups. However, even common sense dictates that an elderly couple is unlikely to be confronted with the same problem as middle-aged patients. For the elderly, lack of family and social support may be far more urgent than in the midlife group. Yet, it must be acknowledged, albeit based on limited data, that family and couples problems in the pain population among the elderly are often somber and require intervention. In our own investigations, we found extraordinary levels of family dysfunction among college students with or without pain. This may suggest that parents of these children are entering midlife and may be especially vulnerable.

We came to the conclusion that much of the so-called nonclinical pain is to be found in all age groups. Perhaps, it is a misnomer to call these pain conditions nonclinical on the grounds that on close scrutiny we found evidence of suffering and perhaps undermanagement of pain in these individuals. This was especially evident at the two ends of the adulthood lifespan. Young adults and the elderly, in our estimation, sometimes fall prey to being overlooked or the seriousness of their pain underestimated. In our own research with both groups, we were constantly astonished to find subsamples of university students who frequently reported pain (which would fall into the category of chronic pain according to IASP definition), and who had the benefit of mostly nonnarcotic analgesics. This group was totally unaware of pain clinics, and their care providers did not see fit to refer them either to medical specialists or to the pain clinics. The elderly and the young adult seemed to share another rather unexpected attitude. Certain kinds of pains were accepted by both as "normal" for their age groups: joint pain and pain in general for the elderly, and cramps, stomach pain, headaches, and even back pain for the young adults.

Two points are noteworthy. First, that variability in health status is perhaps at its maximum with the elderly. Healthy 80 plus persons abound in our society, whereas many do not survive to enjoy their 80th birthday, and still many others live with chronic and debilitating disorders. In other words, it is somewhat misleading to generalize about the health of the elderly population. The second point pertains to young adults. These individuals are generally in the prime of their health, and it stands to reason that they may be inclined to overlook their aches and pains or underestimate their seriousness, which may also be the case with their health care professionals.

It may be instructive to explore the clinical implications for the attitudes of both groups. The fact that the elderly tend to normalize their pain is well established. Caregivers also minimize or normalize pain in the elderly. Ageism remains a fact of life. This adds urgency to the need to recognize and treat pain in the elderly with the same combination of physical and psychological therapies available to the pain clinic population.

The proposition is somewhat more complex with the young adults. Our research pointed up that university students, despite chronic pain, remain more or less functional in their educational pursuit. They give little in the way of outward signs of pain and suffering. They may tend to underplay their aches and pain when visiting their family physicians, and this mitigates against an adequate diagnostic workup. What proportion of these young pain sufferers assume chronic pain status is not well established. Nevertheless, certain kinds of pain, such as headaches, tend to persist well into the middle years and beyond. Is it conceivable that if young patients are taught proper methods of self-management that complements analgesic treatment, that some may avoid falling prey to chronic pain? Again, the answer is largely unknown.

The question of psychopathology and chronic pain as it relates to different life stages merits attention. With the middle-aged pain clinic population, depression has emerged as a relatively common clinical condition. The debate about the nature of this depression, while continuing, seems to be moving in the direction of consensus. While depression is an inherent part of chronic pain for some, for others the depression is dysthymic, and for still others depression is a comorbid condition. Nevertheless, depression of one kind or another is a common finding in the middle-aged chronic pain population. Other psychiatric disorders in this age group of pain patients have not been investigated to the same level of scrutiny as depression. The incidence and prevalence of somatoform disorders in this population, for instance, are not as well researched as is depression.

With our extensive work on pain in college students, psychopathology in general and depression in particular were far less pronounced than in the pain clinic population. Reasons for this finding were far from self-evident. It may be reasonable to assume that university students are a well-functioning group or that those who participated in our studies were less likely to evidence depression and other kinds of psychiatric disorders. Yet, we did find evidence of depression in individuals in our samples of students, many of whom were untreated either for pain or depression. In one study in particular, which investigated association between childhood abuse and chronic pain, we found several individuals with varying degrees of psychopathology.

The problem of psychopathology and chronic pain in the elderly population is particularly thorny. While depression and somatoform disorders are not uncommon in the elderly, they are not as readily recognized as in their younger counterparts. The reasons are complex for this state of affairs. One plausible and practical explanation is that most pain conditions in the elderly are associated with well-known medical conditions and for that reason psychiatric diagnosis is not as readily invoked as with individuals from pain clinic populations for whom medical diagnosis often is a question mark.

Another plausible reason is that both pain and depression tend to be viewed as normally occurring phenomena in the elderly. Depression as a result of many losses is seen as a "normal" reaction by practitioners and patients alike. So is pain. Old age simply means having to live with one or more painful chronic conditions. In these circumstances, pain is viewed as very much an issue of life stage and loses some of the social arguments for active treatment. Fortunately, given the interest in this topic in the scientific literature, some of the stereotypical perspectives are losing ground, and the hope is that the elderly chronic pain sufferer will receive the same kind of attention as the younger pain clinic patients.

We have tentative evidence that social support in the way of social and recreational facilities tend to keep elderly chronic pain suffers healthy. In fact, our own studies revealed an astonishing fact that elderly persons involved in active community and recreational activities viewed themselves as "healthy" despite the presence of chronic pain problems. Some of the distress associated with life transitions in old age, such as loss of loved ones, loss of health, and social isolation, were substantially buffered by their involvement in meaningful friendships and activities.

In relation to young adults, we strongly advocate establishment of health-oriented clinics in universities and colleges to provide courses in self-management of chronic pain problems in students. Pain problems, indeed, of a chronic nature, abound in this population. We concluded from our research that this population was not gaining from the mounting knowledge about psychological approaches to pain management. By and large, students were only treated symptomatically with analgesics. Active intervention with this group may have the potential of preventing long-term chronicity.

In relation to the middle-aged patients who crowd our pain clinics, the issue of life transition could be central in our efforts to appreciate the social, psychological, and familial elements that could be shaping their responses to chronic pain. Life events associated with mid-life are many and varied, and these events have the capacity of generating high levels of stress, and indeed there is tentative evidence to suggest an association between negative life events and the onset of chronic pain disorders.

For the pain clinic population, which is mostly middle-aged, life transition issues are critical to the overall understanding of the patient. This phase, as described earlier, is widely recognized as probably just as troublesome as adolescence. The central feature of the mid-life transition is the preparation for entering old age and a redefinition of one's identity. The point of concern is how the altered perception of oneself combined with considerable change in the social environment of a middle-aged patient influences his or her response to the emergence of a chronic pain problem and what motivates him or her to seek some kind of accommodation to cope with this new reality.

Finally, we want to reiterate our general belief that by adding the dimension of the life stage of the patient, we broaden the base of our understanding of the patient. At the risk of repeating, life events are closely allied with life stages and we are just beginning to fully appreciate the significance of life events. Our attitudes and outlooks are also products, to some extent, of our life stage. Without an understanding of these attitudes, we could not begin to explain the apparent apathy on the part of many elderly to their pain conditions or the unwillingness to accept a benign pain condition by a middle-aged or a younger patient. Seemingly, pain and disability for a younger patient carries greater potential losses than for an elderly person. Life transition theories provide us with the analytical tool to analyze these problems.

What we have proposed in this volume is that a certain level of awareness of life transition issues combined with an appreciation of social and family factors can only improve the quality of care of our patients. This is a laudable goal in itself. In reviewing the pain literature across the lifespan from late adolescence to the oldest-old in the elderly, there are some additional observations that can be entertained that would be less evident in looking at and working with specific age cohorts only. If one takes the theoretical position that pain has at least three components, then an understanding of pain necessitates analysis of all three as well as the interaction among them. First, there is a biological basis of etiology for pain, ranging from genetic vulnerability, to a neurochemical basis to a specific disease or injury. Second, there is an individual psychological component to pain composed of factors ranging from perception, cognitive appraisal, affective context, and past experience to the presence of psychopathology. Last, there are social variables that impact on pain behaviors ranging from environmental contingencies to pain, family context including modeling of pain behaviors, to life events and transition between life stages.

Taking this three-component perspective allows the observation that the most common pain complaints in childhood and adolescence (which are headache and recurrent abdominal pain) tend toward explanations that are more biological and social. On the one hand, the pain literature focuses on explanations that are biological, with an emphasis on medical symptoms and precise diagnosis, with an accompanying supposedly identified biological etiology. Alone, this biological approach has not provided very practical predictive information and explanation. Treatment as well is aimed primarily at symptom relief. The social explanations have investigated principally factors such as secondary gain from familial attention and dysfunctional family environments. Again, the social approach alone has not produced consistent relief for high headache and stomach pain frequencies or severity. The psychological component for these common pains in childhood and adolescence has been minimally researched. This likely is related to two issues. One is that there are serious methodological difficulties in collecting reliable self-report data (the primary source of psychological data) from children and adolescents whose cognitive development is evolving; this is evidenced in that their chronological age is not closely matched to their mental age along multiple dimensions. Thus, only external social observation and medical laboratory information of basic biological data are reliably available for this life stage. A second likely hypothesis is that a further bias has developed implicitly among pain researchers with this age cohort that these individuals are too young to have developed stable psychological patterns of functioning that can significantly influence the prevalence and course of common chronic pains. Interestingly, there is no serious consideration of life transition factors related to the prevalence of pain.

Once again, taking a three-component perspective (biological, psychological, and social) allows different observations about explanations for common pain complaints in young adults. For this age cohort, the biological etiology component would appear to be minimized in the pain research literature, as are the social explanations. Rather, what limited research there is for this age cohort tends to focus on psychological factors as explanatory for incidental pain prevalences that are outside accidental injury or identified disease course. However, our ongoing research investigations with this age group have found repeatedly that the breadth of locations of pain complaints as well as prevalence rates mirror and are remarkedly predictive of common locations and frequencies for chronic pain in middle age along a number of dimensions. Although the prevalence of common pain complaints equals or actually exceeds the rates for all other age cohorts, the severity of the reported pain as well as any accompanying disability tends to be minimal in young adults.

The psychological factors at this point in cognitive development are reliable, easy to assess through self-report, and provide direction into the investigation of somatization disorders, hypercondriasis, and other psychiatric conditions often found to be comorbid with chronic pain. Thus, in our research with young adults, depression and anxiety, although present in individuals with pain complaints, were not typically at the clinical levels found in middle-aged pain clinic patients. From a long-term age perspective, the three components appear to have shifted in their perceived relative importance in the pain literature as to their relative explanatory power regarding pain prevalence and pain behaviors. In the young adult age cohorts as compared to the children and adolescents cohorts, biological laboratory data yield little discriminatory information about pain if not related to injury or disease. In contrast, psychological and to a lesser degree social factors provide the most practical information for diagnosis and treatment. Social information gathered is typically limited to issues like parental health history. Again, there would appear to be a missed opportunity theoretically by not looking at the life events and life transition issues occurring systematically for this age cohort.

Continuing the three-component approach to better understand pain, let us now turn to the life stage of middle age. It is during this age interval that the different theoretical components seem most balanced in their explanatory use in the pain literature. At this point there is even investigation into life transition phenomena and their possible impact via the mediating variable of stress. The literature reviewed involving chronic pain in middle age focused primarily on fibromyalgia. All areas of explanation are still being investigated in this pain disorder because the diagnostical criteria are still being established as to necessary versus sufficient conditions. Thus, biological factors discussed in the literature range from neurochemical abnormalities, genetic vulnerability via sex-specific prevalence rates, to endocrine disorders. From the psychological component there are studies in the literature that associate comorbidity of depression and anxiety to prevalence as well as hypotheses that fibromyalgia is primarily just a new classification of somatization disorder. As mentioned before, there is an active interest in the impact of stress on the onset and course of fibromyalgia, which not only has implications for prevalence but also for treatment programs designed for cure and/or remission only.

In the area of social variables there is research into family factors associated with prevalence as well as life transition features such as changes in health status related to children leaving home, "mid-life crisis," and starting new careers. Some of the factors under investigation may be studied at more than one level, for example, menopause and its possible impact on painfulness to touch can be viewed as a biological component or a social component (role change). Thus, in the pain literature for the middle-aged cohort it would appear that the widest range of theoretical approaches to understanding pain are all under investigation and acknowledgment simultaneously and that there are probably interactions taking place among factors.

We will now look at the elderly using the three-component analysis of explanation of pain prevalence and age cohort. Before reviewing each theoretical component separately, there is a particular phenomenon that needs to be considered in the elderly age cohort. This consideration is that there is strong evidence both in our research and in other studies to suggest that the experiencing of pain and the reporting of pain are not synonymous in this age cohort for significant numbers of individuals. From a biological perspective and the increasing prevalence of specific diseases and disorders of physical deterioration in various domains of functioning, the prevalence of pain complaints is notably lower than expected. Furthermore, in our research, the elderly as an age cohort reported fewer common pains on a comparative (with the exception of joint pains) than all other age cohorts. When this issue has been addressed by detailed interviews in some of our research with the elderly, a typical finding has been that a high proportion of the elderly indicate the presence of pain but had not volunteered the information when filling out general surveys. This suggests some type of response bias is likely operating within this age cohort, distorting actual experiences of pain prevalence. With this important anomaly in mind, let us continue our discussion of pain components in the elderly.

From the biological perspective there has been active investigation in the pain literature on a number of fronts. There is ongoing interest in possible changes in pain sensitivities and thresholds as a function of aging. There are numerous studies as well as our own looking at the impact of mental and physical disorders such as dementia and Alzheimer's on the pain experience. In the psychological aspects of pain relating to the elderly, there also has been increasing research interest. In particular, our research as well as others have looked at the comorbidity between pain and depression and its interaction with memory for pain with institutionalized elderly. If indeed there is a masking of pain in the elderly compared to other age cohorts, it may reflect social variables, such as differences in age cohort expectations, as much as psychological factors, such as denial. Again, social factors are of interest in research with the elderly, since life transition theories often use the elderly as examples in portraying the impact of pain as leading to an examination of issues surrounding death and dying.

If we try to sum up our observations from our work with various age groups as well as relate our experiences with the pain literature, we can conclude that pain prevalence changes in relation to age groups. In children and adolescence, the biological and social components seem to dominate the research in looking for explanations relating to prevalence. With the life transition to young adulthood, there appears to be a shift in the pain research that minimizes biological and social factors relative to the psychological component. Progressively, as the next life transition evolves into middle age, there seems to be a broadening of the pain literature into a search for explaining the prevalence of chronic pain using not only a biological, psychological, and social perspective, but more investigations of interactions as well. This is understandable given the concentration of middle-aged individuals attending pain clinics. And as the life transition for many continues into the elderly years, there is again a shift in research focus toward biological explanations for pain prevalence, with collateral interest in social factors with a minimizing of the individual psychological component. This overview of course reflects very general observations drawn from our work both clinically and as research investigators and can be shown to be inaccurate in many specific instances. However, there are many self-evident aspects to this long-term analysis and speculation, so that even if it is in serious error, it will hopefully be provocative and give impetus to the development of a better overview.

References

Ahern, D., Adams, A., & Follick, M. (1985). Emotional and marital disturbance in spouses of chronic low-back pain patients. *Clinical Journal of Pain, 1*, 69–74.

Alfici, S., Seigal, M., & Landau, M. (1989). Primary fibromyalgia syndrome, a variant of depressive disorder? *Psychotherapy and Psychosomatics, 51*, 156–161.

Alfven, G. (1993). The covariation of common psychosomatic symptoms among children from socioeconomically differing areas: An epidemiological study. *Acta Paediatrica Scandinavica, 00*, 000–000.

Ambepitiya, G., Roberts, M., Ranjadayalan, K., & Tallis, R. (1994). Silent exertional myocardial ischemia in the elderly: A quantitative analysis of anginal perceptual threshold and the influence of autonomic function. *Journal of the American Geriatrics Society, 42*(7), 732–737.

American Psychiatric Association. (1987). *Diagnostic and statistical manual of mental disorders* (3rd ed., rev.). Washington, DC: Author.

American Psychiatric Association. (1994). *Diagnostic and statistical manual of mental disorders* (4th ed.). Washington, DC: Author.

Amodeo, M. (1990). Treating the late life alcoholic: Guidelines for working through denial integrating individual, family and group approaches. *Journal of Geriatric Psychiatry, 23*, 91–105.

Anch, A. M., Lue, F. A., McLean, A. N., & Moldofsky, H. (1991). Sleep physiology and psychological aspects of the fibrositis (fibromyalgia) syndrome. *Canadian Journal of Psychology, 45*(2), 179–184.

Anderson, C., & Arnoult, L. (1989). An examination of perceived control, humor, irrational beliefs, and positive stress as moderators of the relation between negative stress and health. *Basic and Applied Social Psychology, 10*, 101–117.

Andersson, G., Fasth, A., Andersson, J., & Berglund, G. (1987). Incidence and prevalence of juvenile chronic arthritis: A population survey. *Annals of Rheumatic Diseases, 46*, 277–281.

Andersson, H. (1994). The epidemiology of chronic pain in a Swedish rural area. Special Issue: Proceedings of chronic pain in society. *Quality of Life Research,* 3(Suppl. 1), S19–S26.

Apley, J. (1975). *The child with abdominal pain.* London: Blackwell Scientific Publications.

Apley, J. & Hale, B. (1973). Children with abdominal pain: How do they grow up? *British Medical Journal, 3*, 7–9.

Arling, G. (1987). Strain, social support, and distress in old age. *Journal of Gerontology, 42*, 107–113.

Arnold, K., & McKenry, P. (1986). Divorce and the mid-life transition: Some preliminary findings. *Journal of Divorce, 9*, 55–63.

Atkinson, J., Slater, M., Grant, I., & Patterson, T. (1988). Depressed mood in chronic low-back pain: Relationship with stressful life events. *Pain, 35*, 47–55.

Baldwin, B. (1991). The outcome of depression in old age. *International Journal of Geriatric Psychiatry, 6*, 395–400.

Bankoff, E. (1994). Women in psychotherapy: Their life circumstances in treatment needs. *Psychotherapy, 31*, 610–619.

Banks, S., & Kerns, R. (1996). Explaining high rates of depression in chronic pain: A diathesis–stress framework. *Psychological Bulletin, 119*, 95–110.

Barr, R. (1983). Recurrent abdominal pain. In: M. D. Levine, W. Corey, A. Crocker, & R. Gross (Eds.), *Developmental behavioral pediatrics* (pp. 521–528). Philadelphia: Saunders.

Barrows, D. (1995). Functional capacity evaluations of persons with chronic fatigue immune dysfunction syndrome. *American Journal of Occupational Therapy, 49*, 327–337.

Barsky, A. (1993). The diagnosis and management of hypochondriacal concerns in the elderly. Scientific Meeting of the Boston Society for Gerontologic Psychiatry (1992, Boston, Massachusetts). *Journal of Geriatric Psychiatry, 26*, 129–141.

Basolo-Kunzer, M., Diamond, S., Maliszewski, M., Weyerman, M., & Reed. (1991). Chronic headache patients' marital and family adjustment. *Issues in Mental Health Nursing, 12*, 133–148.

Bates, M. S., Edwards, W. T., & Anderson, K. (1993). Ethnocultural influences on variations in chronic pain perception. *Pain, 52*(1), 101–112.

Baumstark, K., & Buckelew, S. (1992). Fibromyalgia: Clinical signs, research findings, treatment implications, and future directions. *Annals of Behavioral Medicine, 14*, 282–291.

Bayer, A. J. (1988). Presentation and management of myocardial infarction in the elderly. *British Journal of Hospital Medicine, 40*, 300–314.

Bayer, T. L., Baer, P. F., & Early, C. (1991). Situational and psychophysiological factors in psychologically induced pain. *Pain, 44*(1), 45–50.

Beaulieu, E., & Karpinsky, J. (1981). Group treatment of elderly with ill spouses. *Casework, 62*, 551–557.

Beck, A., & Beamesdefer, A. (1974). Assessment of depression. In: P. Pichot (Ed.), *Psychological assessment in psychopharmacological psychiatry* (pp. 151–169). Basel: Krager.

Beckham, K., & Giordano, J. (1986). Illness and impairment in elderly couples: Implications for marital therapy. *Journal of Applied Family and Child Studies, 35*, 257–264.

Belli, R. (1989). Influences of misleading postevent information: Misinformation interference and acceptance. *Journal of Experimental Psychology: General, 118*, 72–85.

Benjamin, S., Barnes, D., Berger, S., & Clarke, I. (1988). The relationship of chronic pain, mental illness, and organic disorders. *Pain, 32*, 185–195.

Benjamin, S., Mawer, J., & Lennon, S. (1992). The knowledge and beliefs of family care givers about chronic pain patients. *Journal of Psychosomatic Research, 36*, 211–217.

Berger, A., Knutson, J., Mehm, J., & Perkins, K. (1988). The self-report of punitive childhood experiences of young adults and adolescents. *Child Abuse and Neglect, 12*, 251–262.

Bernstein, G. (1991). Comorbidity and severity of anxiety and depressive disorders in a clinic sample. *Journal of the American Academy of Child and Adolescent Psychiatry, 30*(1), 43–50.

Billie, B. (1962). Migraine in schoolchildren. *Acta Pediatrica Scandinavica, Suppl. 51,* 1–151.

Bishop, D., Epstein, N., Keitner, G., Miller, I., & Srinivasan, S. (1986). Stroke: Morale, family functioning, health status, and functional capacity. *Archives of Physical and Rehabilitation Medicine, 67,* 84–87.

Blotcky, A. (1981). Family functioning and physical health: An exploratory study with practical implications. *Family Therapy, 8,* 197–202.

Blumer, D., & Heilbronn, M. (1982). Chronic pain as a variant of depressive disease: The pain prone disorder. *Journal of Nervous and Mental Disorders, 170,* 381–406.

Bohr, T. (1995). Fibromyalgia syndrome and myofascial pain syndrome: Do they exist? Special Issue: Malingering and conversion reactions. *Neurologic Clinics, 13,* 365–384.

Boissevain, M., & McCain, G. (1991a). Toward an integrated understanding of fibromyalgia syndrome: I. Medical and pathophysiological aspects. *Pain, 45,* 227–238.

Boissevain, M., & McCain, G. (1991b). Toward an integrated understanding of fibromyalgia syndrome. II. Psychological and phenomenological aspects. *Pain, 45,* 239–248.

Bonica, J. J. (1977). Basic principles in the management of chronic pain. *Archives of Surgery, 112,* 783–788.

Bonica, J. J. (1990). Evolution and current status of pain programs. *Journal of Pain and Symptom Management, 5*(6), 368–374.

Boyer, W. (1992). Potential indications for the selective serotonin reuptake inhibitors. *International Clinical Psychopharmacology, 6*(Suppl. 5), 5–12.

Bradley, L., Richter, J., Scarinci, I., & Schan, C. (1992). Psychosocial and psychophysical assessments of patients with unexplained chest pain. *American Journal of Medicine, 92,* 65S–73S.

Brattberg, G. (1994). The incidence of back pain and headache among Swedish school children. *Quality of Life Research: An International Journal of Quality of Life Aspects of Treatment, Care, and Rehabilitation, 3*(Suppl. 1), 27–31.

Brattberg, G., Parker, M. G., & Thorslund, M. (1997). A longitudinal study of pain: Reported pain from middle age to old age. *Clinical Journal of Pain, 13*(2), 144–149.

Brennan, P., & Moos, R. (1990). Life stressors, social resources, and late-life drinking. *Psychology and Aging, 5,* 491–501.

Brim, O. (1976). Theories of the male mid-life crisis. *Counselling Psychologist, 6,* 2–9.

Bromberger, J., & Matthews, K. (1994). Employment status and depressive symptoms in middle-aged women: A longitudinal investigation. *American Journal of Public Health, 84,* 202–206.

Bryant, R. A. (1993). Memory for pain and affect in chronic pain patients. *Pain, 54*(3), 347–351.

Buckelew, S., Parker, J., Keefe, F., Deuser, W., Crews, T., Conway, R., Kay, D., & Hewett, J. (1994). Self-efficacy and pain behaviour among subjects with fibromyalgia. *Pain, 59,* 377–384.

Buelow, G. (1995). Comparing students from substance abusing and dysfunctional families: Implications for counselling. *Journal of Counselling and Development, 73,* 327–330.

Buelow, S., & Buelow, G. (1995). Gender differences in late adolescents' substance abuse and family role development. *Journal of Child Adolescent Substance Abuse, 4*, 27–38.

Bugliosi, T., Meloy, T., & Vukov, L. (1990). Acute abdominal pain in the elderly. *Annals of Emergency Medicine, 19*, 1383–1386.

Bunce, S., Larsen, R., & Peterson, C. (1995). Life after trauma: Personality and daily life experience of traumatized people. *Journal of Personality, 63*, 165–188.

Bunnett, N. (1975). Parental financial support and the financial and family problems of college freshman. *Journal of College Student Personnel, 16*, 145–148.

Buskist, W., & Gerbing, D. (1990). *Psychology: Boundaries and frontiers.* Glenview, IL: Scott, Foresman/Little, Brown Higher Education.

Byrne, P. (1984). Psychiatric morbidity in a gynecology clinic: An epidemiological survey. *British Journal of Psychiatry, 144*, 28–34.

Cantril, H. (1964). A fresh look at the human design. *Journal of Individual Psychology, 20*, 129–136.

Carpenter, J. (1994). Older adults in primary health care in the UK: An exploration of the relevance of family therapy. *Family Systems and Medicine, 12*, 133–148.

Cathey, M., Wolfe, F., & Kleinheksel, S. (1988). Functional ability and work status in patients with fibromyalgia. *Arthritis Care and Research, 1*, 85–98.

Caudill, M. (1995). *Managing pain before it manages you.* New York: Guilford.

Chakour, M. C., Gibson, S. J., Bradbeer, M., & Helme, R. D. (1996). The effect of age on A delta and C fibre thermal pain perception. *Pain, 64*(1), 143–152.

Chaney, J., & Peterson, L. (1989). Family variables and disease management in juvenile rheumatoid arthritis. *Journal of Pediatric Psychology, 14*, 389–403.

Chard, M., Hazleman, B., King, R., & Reiss, B. (1991). Shoulder disorders in the elderly: A community survey. *Arthritis and Rheumatism, 34*, 766–769.

Chrischilles, E., Lemke, J., Wallace, R., & Drube, G. (1990). Prevalence and characteristics of multiple analgesic drug use in an elderly study group. *Journal of the American Geriatrics Society, 38*, 979–984.

Christiano, M. (1982). Health care of children: A continuing struggle. *Early Child Development and Care, 8*, 45–52.

Christianson, S. A., & Loftus, E. F. (1990). Some characteristics of people's traumatic memories. *Bulletin of the Psychonomic Society, 28*(3), 195–198.

Chun, D., Turner, J., & Romano, J. (1993). Children of chronic patients: Risk factors for maladjustment. *Pain, 52*, 311–317.

Ciernia, J. (1985). Death concern and businessmen's mid-life crisis. *Psychological Reports, 56*, 83–87.

Coche, J., & Coche, E. (1986). Leaving the institutional setting to enter private practice: A mid-life crisis resolution. *Private Practice, 4*, 43–50.

Cohen, L., Simons, R., Rose, S., & McGowan, J. (1986). Relationships among negative life events, physiological reactivity, and health symptomatology. *Journal of Human Stress, 12*, 142–148.

Cohen, M., Billig, N., Lipson, S., & Rosenthal, A. (1990). Medical correlates of agitation in nursing home residents. *Gerontology, 36*, 150–158.

Conway, M. (1990). On bias in autobiographical recall: Retrospective adjustment following disconfirmed expectations. *Journal of Social Psychology, 130*, 183–189.

Cook, A., & Thomas, M. (1994). Pain and the use of health services among the elderly. *Journal of Aging and Health, 6*, 155–172.

Costa, P. (1986). Cross-sectional studies of personality in a national sample: ii. Stability of neuroticism, extraversion and openness. *Psychology and Aging, 1*, 144–149.

Craig, K. (1978). Social modelling influences on pain. In: R. A. Sternbach (Ed.), *The psychology of pain*. New York: Raven Press.

Craik, F. I. (1971). Age differences in recognition memory. *Quarterly Journal of Experimental Psychology, 23*(3), 316–323.

Creed, F., Murphy, S., & Jayson, M. (1990). Measurement of psychiatric disorder I rheumatoid arthritis. *Journal of Psychosomatic Research, 34*, 79–87.

Cronan, T., Shaw, W., Gallagher, R., & Weisman, M. (1995). Predicting health care use among older osteoarthritis patients in an HMO. *Arthritis Care and Research, 8*, 66–72.

Crook, J., Rideout, E., & Browne, G. (1984). The prevalence of pain complaints in a general population. *Pain, 18*, 299–314.

Crossley, R. (1982). Hospital admissions for abnormal pain in childhood. *Journal of the Royal Society of Medicine, 75*, 772–776.

Cutler, S. J., & Grams, A. E. (1988). Correlates of self-reported everyday memory complaints. *Journal of Gerontology, 43*, 582–590.

Dalsgaard-Nielsen, T., Enberg-Pedersen, H., & Holm, H. (1970). Clinical and statistical investigations of the epidemiology of migraine. *Danish Medical Bulletin, 17*, 138–148.

Danilov, Y., & Selivra, E. (1990). The problem of evaluation of the family interrelationships and the efficacy of psychotherapy for elderly patients. *Trudy Leningradskogo Nauchno Issledovatel' skogo Psikhonevrologicheskogo Instituta im V M Bekhtereva, 125*, 97–103.

Davis, G., Cortez, C., & Rubin, B. (1990). Pain management in the older adult with rheumatoid arthritis or osteoarthritis. *Arthritis Care and Research, 3*, 27–131.

deBenedittis, G., & Lorenzetti, A. (1992). Minor stressful life events (daily hassles) in chronic primary headache: Relationship with MMPI personality patterns. *Headache, 32*, 330–334.

deBenedittis, G., Lorenzetti, A., & Pieri, A. (1990). The role of life events in the onset of primary headaches. *Pain, 40*, 65–75.

deGrace, G., Joshi, P., Pelletier, R., & Beaupre, C. (1994). Consequences psychologiques de la retraite en fonction du sexex et du niveau occupationnel anterieur [Psychological consequences of retirement as a function of sex an prior occupation level]. *Canadian Journal of Aging, 13*, 149–168.

Demlow, L., Laing, M., & Eaton, H. (1986). Impact of chronic arthritis on the elderly. *Clinics in Rheumatic Disease, 12*, 329–336.

Deubner, D. (1977). An epidemiological study of migraine and headache in 10–20 year olds. *Headache, 17*, 173–180.

Diedricks, M. (1995). The social support of students during transition from school to university. *South African Journal of Psychology, 25*, 122–126.

Douglas, D., Suurmeijer, T., Kroll, B., & Sanderman, R. (1994). Social support, social disability, and psychological well being in rheumatoid arthritis. *Arthritis Care and Research, 7*(1), 10–15.

Duckitt, J. (1983). Psychological factors related to subjective health perception among elderly women. *Humanities Journal for Research in the Human Subjects, 9*, 441–449.

Duckitt, J., & Broll, T. (1982). Life event stress, social support and health. *Humanities Journal for Research in the Human Sciences, 8*, 377–383.

Dunne, F., & Dunne, C. (1995). Fibromyalgia syndrome and psychiatric disorder. *British Journal of Hospital Medicine, 54*, 194–197.

Dunn-Geier, B., McGrath, P., Roucke, B., & D'Astous, J. (1986). Adolescent chronic pain. The ability to cope. *Pain, 26*, 23–32.

Dura, J., & Beck, S. (1988). A comparison of family function when mothers have chronic pain. *Pain, 35*, 79–89.

Dworkin, S., Von Korff, M., & LeResche, L. (1992). Epidemiologic studies of chronic pain: A dynamic–ecologic perspective. *Annals of Behavioral Medicine, 14*, 3–11.

Edwards, A. J. (1994). When memory fails: Helping the Alzheimer's and dementia patient. New York: Plenum Press.

Edwards, P., Zeichner, A., Kuczmierczyk, A., & Boczkowski, J. (1985). Familial pain models: The relationship between family history of pain and current pain experience. *Pain, 21*, 379–384.

Egle, U. (1992). The chronic benign pain syndrome: Diagnostic subgroups, screening parameters, biographical disposition [German]. *Psychotherapie, Psychosomatik, Medizinische Psychologie, 42*, 261–272.

Eich, E., Reeves, J. L., Jaeger, B., Graff-Radford, S. B. (1985). Memory for pain: Relation between past and present pain intensity. *Pain, 23*(4), 375–380.

Eisendrath, S. (1995). Psychiatric aspects of chronic pain. *Neurology, 45*(Suppl. 9), s26–s34.

Eiser, C., & Berrenberg, J. (1995). Assessing the impact of chronic disease on the relationship between parents and their adolescents. *Journal of Psychosomatic Research, 39*, 109–114.

Ellertsen, B., Vaeroy, H., Endresen, F., & Forre. (1991). MMPI in fibromyalgia and local nonspecific myalgia. *New Trends in Experimental and Clinical Psychiatry, 7*(2), 53–62.

El-Rufaie, O., & Absood, G. (1993). Minor psychiatric morbidity in primary care: Prevalence, nature and severity. *International Journal of Social Psychiatry, 39*, 159–166.

Engel, G. (1959). "Psychogenic" pain and the pain-prone patient. *American Journal of Medicine, 26*, 899–918.

Epstein, N. B., Bishop, D., Ryan, C., Miller, I., & Keitner, G. I. *The McMaster Model: View of health family functioning normal family processes* (2nd ed.). New York: Guilford Press.

Ercolani, M., Trombini, G., Chattat, R., Cervini, C., et al. (1994). Fibromyalgia syndrome: Depression and abnormal illness behavior: Multicenter investigation. *Psychotherapy and Psychosomatics, 61*(3–4), 178–186.

Erikson, E. (1960). *Identity and the life cycle.* New York: Norton.

Erikson, E. (1980). *Identity and the life cycle: A reissue.* New York: Norton.

Estlander, A., Takala, E., & Verkasalo, M. (1995). Assessment of depression in chronic musculoskeletal pain patients. *Clinical Journal of Pain, 11*, 194–200.

Evans, P., Pitts, M., & Smith, K. (1988). Minor infection, minor life events and the four day desirability dip. *Journal of Psychosomatic Research, 32*, 533–539.

Fabrega, H., & Miller, B. (1995). Adolescent psychiatry as a product of modern Anglo-American society. *Social Science and Medicine, 40*, 881–894.

Falger, P. (1983). Pathogenic life changes in middle adulthood and coronary heart disease: A life span developmental perspective. *International Journal of Human Development and Aging, 16*, 7–27.

Farrar, D., Locke, S., & Kantrowitz, F. (1995). Chronic fatigue syndrome 1: Etiology and pathogenesis. *Behavioural Medicine, 21*, 5–16.

Faucett, J., & Levine, J. (1991). The contribution of interpersonal conflict to chronic pain in the presence of absence or organic pathology. *Pain, 44*, 35–43.

Ferrell, B. A., Ferrell, B. R., & Osterweil, D. (1990). Pain in the nursing home. *Journal of the American Geriatric Society, 38*(4), 401–404.

Ferrell, B. A., Ferrell, B. R., & Rivera, L. (1995). Pain in cognitively impaired nursing home patients. *Journal of Pain and Symptom Management, 10*(8), 591–598.

Ferrin, R. L., Edelstein, S. L., & Barrett-Conner, E. (1994). Factors associated with health behavior change among residents 50 to 96 years of age in Rancho Benardo, California. *American Journal of Preventive Medicine, 10*(1), 26–30.

Feuerstein, M., Sult, S., & Houle, M. (1985). Environmental stressors and chronic low back pain: Life events, family and work environment. *Pain, 22*, 295–307.

Field, D., Minkler, M., Falk, F., & Leino, V. (1993). Influence of health on family contacts and family feelings in advanced old age: A longitudinal study. *Journal of Gerontology, 48*, 18–28.

Finney, J., & Bonner, M. (1992). The influence of behavioral family intervention on the health of chronically ill children. *Behavior Change, 9*, 157–170.

Fitzpatrick, R., Newman, S., Lamb, R., & Shipley, M. (1988). Social relationships and psychological well-being in rheumatoid arthritis. *Social Science and Medicine, 27*, 399–403.

Flett, G., Blankstein, K., Kirk, R., Hicken, J., & Watson, M. (1995). Social support and help seeking in daily hassles versus major life events stress. *Journal of Applied Social Psychology, 25*, 279–294.

Flor, H., Turk, D., & Rudy, T. (1987). Pain and families II: Assessment and treatment. *Pain, 30*, 29–54.

Flor, H., Turk, D., & Rudy, T. (1989). Relationship of pain impact and significant other reinforcement of pain behaviours: The mediating role of gender, marital status and marital satisfaction. *Pain, 38*, 45–50.

Flor, H., Turk, D., & Scholz, B. (1987). Impact of chronic pain on the spouse: Marital, emotional and physical consequences. *Journal of Psychosomatic Research, 31*, 63–71.

Floyd, F., Haynes, S., Doll, E., Winemiller, D., & Lemsky, C. (1992). Assessing retirement satisfaction and perceptions of retirement experience. *Psychology and Aging, 7*, 609–621.

Folstein, M., et al. (1985). The meaning of cognitive impairment in the elderly. *Journal of the American Geriatrics Society, 33*(4), 228–235.

Folstein, M., Folstein, S., & McHugh, P. (1975). Minimental state. *Journal of Psycholinguistic Research, 12*, 189–198.

Fordyce, W. (1976). *Behavioral methods for chronic pain and illness.* St. Louis: Mosby.

Fordyce, W. E. (1983). Behavioral conditioning concepts in chronic pain. In: J. Bonica, (Ed.), *Advances in pain research* (pp. 781–788). New York: Raven Press.

Fordyce, W. (1993). Effects of marital interaction on chronic pain and disability: Examining the down side of social support: Comment. *Rehabilitation Psychology, 38*, 211–212.

Fowlie, S., Eastwood, M., & Ford, M. (1992). Irritable bowel syndrome: The influence of psychological factors on the symptom complex. *Journal of Psychosomatic Research, 36*, 169–173.

France, R. D. & Urban, B. J. (1991). Cerebrospinal fluid concentrations of beta-endorphin in chronic low back pain patients: Influence of depression and treatment. *Psychosomatics, 32*(1), 72–77.

Frischer, M., Ford, G., & Taylor, R. (1991). Life events and psychological well-being in old age. *Psychology and Health, 5*, 203–219.

Frisoni, G., de Leo, D., Rozzini, R., & Bernardini, M. (1993). Night sleep symptoms in an elderly population and their relation with age, gender, and education. *Clinical Gerontologist, 13*, 51–68.

Fry, P. (1990). A factor analytic investigation of homebound elderly individuals' concerns about death and dying, and their coping responses. *Journal of Clinical Psychology, 46*, 737–748.

Fry, P., & Wong, P. (1991). Pain management training in the elderly: Matching interventions with subjects' coping styles. *Stress Medicine, 7*, 93–98.

Gallo, J., Royall, D., & Anthony, J. (1993). Risk factors for the onset of depression in middle age and later life. *Social Psychiatry and Psychiatric Epidemiology, 28*, 101–108.

Gare, B., & Fasth, A. (1992). Epidemiology of juvenile chronic arthritis in southwestern Sweden: A 5-year prospective study. *Pediatrics, 90*, 950–958.

Garrison, J., & Howe, J. (1976). Community intervention with the elderly: A social network approach. *Journal of the American Geriatric Society, 24*, 329–333.

Gaston-Johansson, F., Gustaffson, M., Felldin, R., & Sanne, H. (1990). A comparative study of feelings, attitudes and behaviors of patients with fibromyalgia and rheumatoid arthritis. *Social Science and Medicine, 31*, 941–947.

Gentili, P., & Francescangeli, M. (1987). Evaluation of some adaptation characteristics in psoriatic arthritis patients. [Italian] *Medicina Psicisomatica, 32*, 315–327.

Gentry, W., Shows, W. D., & Thomas, M. R. (1974). Chronic low back pain: A psychological profile. *Psychosomatics, 15*, 174–177.

Getzel. (1982). Helping elderly couples in crisis. *Social Casework, 63*, 515–521.

Gewanter, H., Roghmann, K., & Barin, J. (1983). The prevalence of juvenile arthritis. *Arthritis and Rheumatology, 26*, 599–603.

Gibson, S., Katz, B., Corran, T., Farrell, M., et al. (1994). Pain in older persons. Special Issue: Disability and rehabilitation in older persons. *Disability and Rehabilitation, 16*, 127–139.

Gibson, S. J., & Helme, R. D. (1995). Age differences in pain perception and report: A review of physiological, psychological, laboratory, and clinical studies. *Pain Reviews, 2*(2), 111–137.

Gilleard, C., Lieberman, S., & Feeler, R. (1992). Family therapy for older adults: A survey of professionals' attitudes. *Journal of Family Therapy, 14*, 413–422.

Goldberg, G., Kerns, R., & Rosenberg, R. (1993). Pain-relevant support as a buffer from depression among chronic pain patients low in instrumental activity. *Clinical Journal of Pain, 9*, 34–40.

Goldstein, M. (1990). The role of mutual support groups and family therapy for caregivers of demented elderly. *Journal of Geriatric Psychiatry, 23*, 117–128.

Goldstein, S., & Birnbaum, F. (1976). Hypochondriasis and the elderly. *Journal of the American Geriatric Society, 24*, 150–154.

Goodenow, C., Reisine, S., & Grady, K. (1990). Quality of social support and associated social and psychological functioning in women with rheumatoid arthritis. *Health Psychology, 9*, 266–284.

Goodman, J., & McGrath, P. (1991). The epidemiology of pain in children and adolescents: A review. *Pain, 46*, 247–264.

Goodnick, P. J., & Sardoral, R. (1993). Psychotropic treatment of chronic fatigue syndrome and related disorders. *Journal of Clinical Psychiatry, 54*(1), 13–20.

Gordino, A. (1983). Researches on the mid-life crisis and the psychology of adult life. [Italian] *Rivista Sperimentale di Freniatria e Medicina Legale della Alienazioni Mentali 107*, 958–976.

Graham, H., Senior, N., Dukes, S., Lazarus, M., et al. (1993). The introduction of family therapy to British general practice. *Family Systems and Medicine, 11*, 363–373.

Grassetto, M., & Varotto, A. Primary fibromyalgia is responsive to S-adenosyl-L-methionine. *Current Therapeutic Research, 55*(7), 797–806.

Green, B., Copeland, J., Dewey, M., Sharma, V., et al. (1994). Factors associated with recovery and recurrence of depression in older people: A prospective study. *International Journal of Geriatric Psychiatry, 9*, 789–795.

Greene, J., Walker, L., Hickson, G., & Thompson, J. (1985). Stressful life events and somatic complaints in adolescents. *Pediatrics, 75*, 19–22.

Greene, R. (1976). A life span approach to understanding parent–child relationships in aging families. *Journal of Psychotherapy and the Family, 5*, 57–69.

Guralnik, J. M., Yanagashita, M., & Schneider, E. I. (1988). Projecting the older population of the United States: Lessons from the past and prospects for the future. *The Milbank Quarterly, 66*, 283–308.

Gutman, D. (1976). Individual adaptation in the middle years: Developmental issues in the masculine mid-life crisis. *Journal of Geriatric Psychiatry, 9*, 41–59.

Hagborg, W. (1992). Prevalence and correlates of self-reported depressive mood among seriously emotionally disturbed adolescents. *Psychological Reports, 70*, 23–26.

Hagglund, K., Deuser, W., Buckelew, S., Hewett, J., et al. (1994). Weather, beliefs about weather, and disease severity among patients with fibromyalgia. *Arthritis Care and Research, 7*, 130–135.

Hagglund, K., Schoop, L., Alberts, K., Cassidy, J., et al. (1995). Predicting pain among children with juvenile rheumatoid arthritis. *Arthritis Care and Research, 8*, 36–42.

Hardy, P. (1995). Pain management in old age. *Reviews in Clinical Gerontology, 5*, 259–273.

Harkappa, K. (1992). Psychosocial factors as predictors for early retirement in patients with chronic low back pain. *Journal of Psychosomatic Research, 36*, 553–559.

Harkins, S., & Chapman, C. (1976). Detection and decision factors in pain perception in young and elderly men. *Pain, 2*, 253–264.

Harkins, S., & Chapman, C. (1977). The perception of induced dental pain in young and elderly women. *Journal of Gerontology, 32*, 428–435.

Harkins, S., Lagua, B., Price, D., & Small, R. E. (1995). Geriatric pain. In: R. Roy (Ed.), *Chronic pain in old age* (pp. 127–160).

Harkins, S. W. (1988). Pain in the elderly. In: R. Dubner, G. F. Gebhart, & M. R. Bond (Eds.), *Proceedings of the Vth World Congress on Pain* (pp. 355–367). Amsterdam: Elsevier Science Publishers.

Harkins, S. W., & Price, D. D. (1997). Assessment of pain in the elderly. In: D. Turk & R. Melzack (Eds.), *Handbook of pain assessment* (pp. 315–331).

Hasher, L., & Zacks, R. (1988). Working memory, comprehension, and aging: A review and a new view. In: Gordon H. Bower (Ed.), *The psychology of learning and motivation, Volume 2: Advances in research and theory* (pp. 193–225). San Diego: Academic Press.

Haythornthwaite, J., Sieber, W., & Kerns, R. (1991). Depression and the chronic pain experience. *Pain, 46*, 177–184.

Hedlund, B., & Ebersole, P. (1983). A test of Levinson's mid-life evaluation. *Journal of Genetic Psychology, 143*, 189–192.

Helme, R., & Gibson, S. (1996). *Pain in the elderly.* Seattle, WA: International Association of the Society of Pain Press.

Helme, R., Gibson, S., & Farrell, M. (1996). *The influence of social factors on the chronic pain experience in older people.* Abstracts (s19). Vancouver, Canada: World Congress of the International Association for the Study of Pain.

Helson, R., & Wink, P. (1992). Personality change in women from the early 40's to the early 50's. *Psychology and Aging, 7,* 46–55.

Henriksson, C. (1995). Living with continuous muscular pain—Patient perspectives: I. Encounters and consequences. *Scandinavian Journal of Caring Sciences, 9,* 67–76.

Henriksson, C., Gundmark, I., Bengtsson, A., & Ek, A. (1992). Living with fibromyalgia: Consequences for everyday life. *The Clinical Journal of Pain, 8,* 138–144.

Herr, K., & Mobily, P. (1991). Complexities of pain assessment in the elderly: Clinical considerations. *Journal of Gerontology Nursing, 17,* 12–19.

Heuer, F., & Reisberg, D. (1990). Vivid memories of emotional events: The accuracy of remembered minutiae. *Memory and Cognition, 18,* 496–506.

Higgitt, A. (1992). Dependency on prescribed drugs. *Reviews in Clinical Gerontology, 2*(2), 151–155.

Hill, E., Nord, J., & Blow, F. (1992). Young-adult children of alcoholic parents: Cohesion, adaptability and addiction. *British Journal of Addiction, 87,* 1677–1690.

Hinkle, L. (1961). Ecological observations of the relation of physical illness, mental illness and the social environment. *Journal of Psychomatic Medicine, 23,* 289–297.

Hinkle, L., & Wolfe, H. (1957). The nature of man's adaptation to his total environment and the relation of this to illness. *Archives of Internal Medicine, 99,* 442–460.

Hochberg, M., Linet, M., & Sills, E. (1983). The prevalence and incidence of juvenile rheumatoid arthritis in an urban black population. *American Journal of Public Health, 73,* 1202–1203.

Hodges, K., Kline, J., Barbero, G., & Flanery, R. (1984). Life-events occurring in families of children with recurrent abdominal pain. *Journal of Psychosomatic Research, 28,* 185–188.

Hodgkiss, A. (1997). Rediscovering the psychopathology of chronic pain. *Journal of Psychosomatic Research, 42*(3), 221–224.

Hoekstra, R., Ronhaar, P. K., & Laporte, R. B. (1996). On the boundary between compulsory and voluntary hospitalization. *Psychiatric, 38*(10), 713–722.

Holmes, T., & Rahe, R. (1967). The social readjustment rating scale. *Journal of Psychosomatic Research, 11,* 213–218.

Holroyd, J. (1996). Hypnosis treatment of clinical pain: Understanding why hypnosis is useful. *International Journal of Clinical and Experimental Hypnosis, 44*(1), 33–51.

Huckle, P. (1994). Families and dementia. *International Journal of Geriatric Psychiatry, 9,* 735–741.

Hudgens, A. (1979). Family-oriented treatment of chronic pain. *Journal of Marriage and Family Therapy, 5,* 67–78.

Hughston, G., Christopherson, V., & Bonjean, M. (1989). Aging and family therapy: An introduction. *Journal of Marriage and Family, 46,* 845–852.

Hunter, M., Philips, C., & Rachmar, S. (1979). Memory for pain. *Pain, 6*(1), 35–46.

Huskisson, E. (1983) Visual analog scale. In: R. Melzack (Ed.), *Pain measurement and assessment* (pp. 33–40). New York: Raven Press.

International Association for the Study of Pain Subcommittee on Taxonomy. (1986). *Pain* (Suppl. 3), *0,* 000–000.

Jack, S. (1981). *Current estimates from National Health Interview Survey.* United States Vital and Health Statistics, Series 10, No. 136 (DHHS Publication No. 81-1564). Washington, DC: US Government Printing Office.

Jacox, A., Carr, D. B., & Payne, R. (1994). New clinical practice guidelines for the management of pain in patients with cancer. *New England Journal of Medicine, 330*(9), 651–655.

Jamison, R., & Virts, K. (1990). The influence of chronic support on chronic pain. *Behaviour Research and Therapy, 28,* 283–287.

Jaworski, T. (1993). Juvenile rheumatoid arthritis: Pain-related and psychosocial aspects and their relevance for assessment and treatment. *Arthritis Care and Research, 6,* 187–196.

Jenike, M. (1996). Psychiatric illnesses in the elderly: A review. *Journal of Geriatric Psychiatry and Neurology, 9,* 57–82.

Jenkins, P. (1991). Psychogenic abdominal pain. *General Hospital Psychiatry, 13,* 27–30.

Jensen, J. (1988). Life events in neurologic patients with headache and low back pain in relation to diagnosis and persistence of pain. *Pain, 32,* 47–53.

Jensen, M. P., & Karoly, P. (1997). Comparative self-evaluation and depressive affect among chronic pain patients: An examination of selective evaluation theory. *Cognitive Therapy and Research, 16*(3), 297–308.

Johansson, G., Risberg, J., Rosenhall, U., & Orndahl, G. (1995). Cerebral dysfunction in fibromyalgia: Evidence from regional cerebral blood flow measurements, otoneurological tests and cerebrospinal fluid analysis. *Acta Psychiatrica Scandinavica, 91*(2), 86–94.

Johnson, B., & Theorell, T. (1991). Life events, abdominal pain and depression in peptic ulcer and depressive disorder. *International Journal of Psychosomatics, 38*(Special Issue), 27–32.

Julian, T., McKenry, P., & McKelvey, M. (1992). Components of men's well-being at midlife. *Issues in Mental Health Nursing, 13,* 285–299.

Kaplan, K. H., Goldenberg, D. L., & Galvin-Nadeau, M. (1993). The impact of a mediation-based stress reduction program on fibromyalgia. *General Hospital Psychiatry, 15*(5), 284–289.

Kaplan, G., Barell, V., & Lusky, A. (1988). Subjective state of health and survival in elderly adults. *Journal of Gerontology, 43*(Suppl.), 114–118.

Kaplan, H., & Sadock, B. (1989). *Comprehensive textbook of psychiatry.* Baltimore: Williams & Wilkins.

Katon, W., & Sullivan, M. (1990). Depression and chronic medical illness. *Journal of Clinical Psychiatry, 51*(Suppl.), 3–11.

Katz, I., Parmelee, P., & Streim, J. (1995). Depression in older patients in residential care: Significance of dysphoria and dimensional assessment. *American Journal of Geriatric Psychiatry, 3,* 161–169.

Kausler, D. H., & Wiley, J. G. (1991). Effects of short-term retrieval on adult age differences in long-term recall of actions. *Psychology and Aging, 6*(4), 661–665.

Keller, R. (1994). Psychosomatic syndromes, somatization, and somatoform disorders. *Psychotherapy and Psychosomatics, 61*(1–2), 4–24.

Kerns, R., & Jacob, M. (1992). Assessment of the psychosocial context in the experience of pain. In: D. C. Turk & R. Melzack (Eds.), *Handbook of pain assessment* (pp. 235–256). New York: Guilford.

Kerns, R., & Turk, D. (1984). Chronic pain and depression: Mediating role of the spouse. *Journal of Marriage and Family, 46,* 845–852.

Kerns, R., Haythornthwaite, J., Southwick, S., & Giller, E. (1990). The role of marital interaction in chronic pain and depressive symptoms severity. *Journal of Psychosomatic Research, 34*, 401–408.

Kihlstrom, J., & Harackiewicz, J. (1982). The earliest recollection: A new survey. *Journal of Personality, 50*, 135–148.

King, K., & Hanson, V. (1986). Psychosocial aspects of juvenile rheumatoid arthritis. *Pediatric Clinics of North America, 33*, 1221–1237.

Klages, U. (1991). Life events and irrational attitude in patients with rheumatoid arthritis: Relation to pain, disability and general health condition. *International Journal of Psychosomatics, 38*, 21–26.

Klerman, G. L. (1983). Problems in the definition and diagnosis of depression in the elderly. In: M. Hauge & L. Breslau (Eds.), *Depression in the elderly: Causes, care, consequences* (pp. 119–138). New York: Springer.

Kopp, M., Richter, R., Rainer, J., Kopp-Wilfing, P., et al. (1995). Differences in family functioning between patients with chronic headache and patients with chronic low-back pain. *Pain, 63*, 219–224.

Kosek, E., Ekholm, J., & Hansson, P. (1995). Increased pressure pain sensibility in fibromyalgia patients is located deep to the skin but not restricted to muscle tissue. *Pain, 63*(3), 335–339.

Krag, N., Norregaard, J., Larsen, J., & Danneskiold-Samsoe, B. (1994). A blinded, controlled evaluation of anxiety and depressive symptoms in patients with fibromyalgia, as measured by standardized psychometric interview scales. *Acta Psychiatrica Scandinavica, 89*, 370–375.

Kramlinger, K., Swanson, D., & Maruta, T. (1983). Are patients with chronic pain depressed? *American Journal of Psychiatry, 140*, 747–749.

Kriegsman, D., Penninx, B., & van Eijk, J. (1995). A criterion-based literature survey in the relationship between family support and incidence and course of chronic disease in the elderly. *Family Systems and Medicine, 13*, 39–68.

Kuch, K., Evans, R. J., Watson, P. C., Bubela, C. et al. (1991). Road vehicle accidents and phobias in 60 patients with fibromyalgia. *Journal of Anxiety Disorders, 5*(3), 273–280.

Kuch, K., Cox, B., Evans, R., Watson, P., & Bubela, C. (1993). To what extent do anxiety and depression interact with chronic pain? *Canadian Journal of Psychiatry, 38*, 36–38.

Kunnamo, I., Kallio, P., & Pelkonen, P. (1986). Incidence of arthritis in urban Finnish children. A prospective study. *Arthritis and Rheumatism, 29*, 1232–1238.

Kwentus, J., Harkins, S., Lignon, N., & Silverman, J. (1985). Current concepts of geriatric pain and its treatment. *Geriatrics, 40*, 48–57.

Lautenbacher, S., Rollman, G. B., & McCain, G. A. (1994). Multi-method assessment of experimental and clinical pain in patients with fibromyalgia. *Pain, 59*(1), 45–53.

Lavigne, J., Schulein, M., & Hahn, Y. (1986). Psychological aspects of painful medical conditions in children. II. Personality factors, family characteristics and treatment. *Pain, 27*, 147–169.

LeWall, J. (1981). Conjoint therapy for psychiatric problems in the elderly. *Journal of American Geriatric Society, 29*, 89–91.

La Rue, A., Dessonville, C., & Jarvik, L. F. (1985). Aging and mental disorders. In: J. E. Birren & K. W. Schaie (Eds.), *Handbook of the psychology of aging* (2nd ed., pp. 664–702). New York: Van Nostrand Reinhold.

Ledingham, J., Doherty, S., & Doherty, M. (1993). Primary fibromyalgia syndrome: An outcome study. *British Journal of Rheumatology, 32*, 139–142.

Lee, M. (1989). An ecological view of aging: Luisa's plight. *Journal of the Gerontological Society, Week 14*, 175–190.

Lennon, M., Dohrenwend, B., Zaruta, A., & Marbach, J. (1990). Coping and adaptation to facial pain in contrast to other stressful life events. *Journal of Personality and Social Psychology, 59*, 1040–1050.

Levine, M., & Rappaport, L. (1984). Recurrent abdominal pain in school children: The loneliness of long-distance physician. *Pediatric Clinics of North America, 31*, 969–991.

Levinson, D. (1977). A period in adult psychological development. *Psychiatry, 40*, 99–112.

Levinson, D. (1978). *The seasons of a man's life*. New York: Knopf.

Levkoff, S., Cleary, P., Wetle, T., & Besdine, W. (1988). Illness behavior in the aged: Implications for clinicians. *Journal of the American Geriatrics Society, 36*, 622–629.

Liebman, R., Honig, P., & Berger, H. (1976). An integrated treatment approach for psychogenic pain. *Family Process, 15*, 397–405.

Light, L. L. (1991). Memory and aging: Four hypotheses in search of data. *Annual Review of Psychology, 42*, 333–376.

Lindberg, T. (1994). Recurrent abdominal pain in childhood. *Acta Paediatrica, 83*, 775–776.

Lindsay, P., & Wyckoff, M. (1981). The depression–pain syndrome and its response to antidepressants. *Psychosomatics, 22*, 571–577.

Linet, M., Stewart, W., Celentano, D., Ziegler, D., & Sprecher, M. (1989). An epidemiologic study of headache among adolescents and young adults. *Journal of the American Medical Association, 261*, 2211–2216.

Linton, S. J., & Melin, L. (1982). The accuracy of remembering chronic pain. *Pain, 13*(3), 281–285.

Locke, H., & Wallace, K. (1959). Short marital-adjustment and prediction tests: Their reliability and validity. *Marriage and Family Living, 21*, 251–255.

Loftus, E. F., & Hoffman, H. G. (1989). Misinformation and memory: The creation of new memories. *Journal of Experimental Psychology, 118*, 100–104.

Louis Harris and Associates (1985). *The Nuprin Report*. New York: Author.

Lousberg, R., Schmidt, A. J. M., & Groenman, N. H. (1992). The relationship between spouse solicitousness and pain behaviour: Searching for more experimental evidence. *Pain, 51*, 75–79.

Lundry, L., Sandback, A., & Juul, S. (1990). Recurrent abdominal pain in school children 9–12 years of age. [Danish] *Ugeskruft for Laeger, 152*, 2851–2854.

Luscher, C. (1993). Labor, employment, professions, and retirement: Does retirement precipitate depression in older adults? [German] *Żeitschrift Gerontopsychologie and Psychiatrie, 6*, 39–49.

Madanes, C. (1981). *Strategic family therapy*. San Francisco: Jossey-Bass.

Maes, M., Calabrese, J., Lee, M., & Meltzer, H. (1994). Effects of age on spontaneous cortisolaemia of normal volunteers and depressed patients. *Psychoneuroendocrinology, 19*, 79–84.

Magni, G., Caldieron, C., Rigatti, L., & Merskey, H. (1990). Chronic musculoskeletal pain and depressive symptoms in the general population: An analysis of the 1st National Health and Nutrition Examination Survey data. *Pain, 43*, 299–307.

Manne, S., & Zaruta, A. (1989). Spouse criticism and support: Their association with coping and psychological adjustment among women with rheumatoid arthritis. *Journal of Personality and Social Psychology, 56*, 608–617.

Manners, P., & Diepeveen, D. (1996). Prevalence of juvenile chronic arthritis in a population of 12 year old children in urban Australia. *Pediatrics, 98*, 84–89.

Marbach, J., Lennon, M., & Dohrenwend, B. P. (1988). Candidate risk factors for temporomandibular pain and dysfunction syndrome: Psychosocial, health behavior, physical illness and injury. *Pain, 34*, 139–151.

Martinez, J., Ferraz, M., Fontana, A., & Atra, E. (1995). Psychological aspects of Brazilian women with fibromyalgia. *Journal of Psychosomatic Research, 39*, 167–174.

Martinez, J., Ferraz, M., Sato, E., & Atra, E. (1995). Fibromyalgia versus rheumatoid arthritis: A longitudinal comparison of the quality of life. *Journal of Rheumatology, 22*, 270–274.

Marykuca, S. (1994). *Influences of discipline practices of parents on pain prevalence in university students.* Honors Thesis Department of Psychology, University of Manitoba, Winnipeg, Canada.

Marzinski, L. R. (1991). The tragedy of dementia: Clinically assessing pain in the confused, nonverbal elderly. *Journal of Gerontological Nursing, 17*(6), 25–28.

Matthew, A., & Brown, K. (1987). Retirement as a critical life event: The differential experience of women and men. *Research on Aging, 9*, 548–571.

Mayou, R. (1998). Chest pains, palpitations, and panic. *Journal of Psychosomatic Research, 44*(1), 53–70.

McCorkle, R., Benoliel, J. Q., Donaldson, G., Georgiadou, F., Moinpour, C., & Goodell, B. (1989). A randomized clinical trial of home nursing care for lung cancer patients. *Cancer, 64*, 1375–1382.

McFadyen, A., Broster, G., & Black, D. (1991). The impact of a child psychiatry liaison service on patterns of referral. *British Journal of Psychiatry, 158*, 93–96.

McGinnies, E., & Ward, C. (1980). Better liked than right: Trustworthiness and expertise as factors in credibility. *Personality and Social Psychology Bulletin, 6*, 467–472.

McGrath, P., & Feldman, W. (1986). Clinical approach to recurrent abdominal pain in children. *Developmental and Behavioral Pediatrics, 7*, 56–61.

McGrath, P., & Unruh, A. (1987). *Pain in children and adolescents.* New York: Elsevier.

McGrath, P., Goodman, J., Firestone, P., Shipman, R., & Peters, S. (1983). Recurrent abdominal pain: A psychogenic disorder? *Archives of Diseases of Childhood, 58*, 880– 890.

McGuigan, J. (1995). Attributional style and depression in men receiving treatment for chronic pain. *Journal of Applied Rehabilitation and Counseling, 26*, 21–25.

McNeil, J., & Harsany, M. (1989). An age difference view of depression. Special Issue: Psychology of aging and gerontology. *Canadian Psychology, 30*, 608–615.

Mechanic, D. (1983). Adolescent health and illness behavior. *Journal of Human Stress, 9*, 4–13.

Melanson, P., & Downe-Wamboldt, B. (1995). The stress of life with rheumatoid arthritis as perceived by older adults. *Activities, Adaptation and Aging, 19*, 33–47.

Melding, P. (1991). Is there such a thing as geriatric pain? *Pain, 46*, 119–121.

Mellor, K., & Edelmann, R. (1988). Mobility, social support, loneliness and well-being amongst two groups of old adults. *Personality and Individual Differences, 9*, 1–5.

Merskey, A., & Boyd, D. (1978). Emotional adjustment and chronic pain. *Pain, 5*, 173–178.

Merskey, H. (1996). Plenary session on fibromyalgia: Introduction. *Pain Research and Management, 1*, 41–53.

Meunier, G. (1994). Marital therapy with elderly couple. *Journal of Contemporary Psychotherapy, 24*, 125–129.

Midanik, L., Soghikian, K., Ransom, L., & Tekawa, I. (1995). The effect of retirement on mental health behaviors: The Kaiser Permanent Retirement Study. *Journal of Gerontology, 50B*, s59–s61.

Mielants, H., Veys, E., Maertens, M., Goemaere, S., et al. (1993). Prevalence of inflammatory rheumatic diseases in an adolescent urban student population. *Clinical and Experimental Rheumatology, 11*, 563–567.

Mikail, S., & von Bayer, C. (1990). Pain, somatic focus and emotional adjustment in children of chronic headache sufferers and controls. *Social Science and Medicine, 31*, 51–59.

Miller, P. F., Sheps, D., Bragdon, E., Herbst, M., Dalton, J. L., Hindeliter, A. L., Koch, G. S., Mairiner, W., & Ekelund, L. (1990). Aging and pain perception in ischemic heart disease. *American Heart Journal, 120*, 22–30.

Minuchim, S. (1974). *Families and family therapy.* Cambridge, MA: Harvard University Press.

Mirowsky, J., & Ross, C. (1992). Age and depression. *Journal of Health and Social behavior, 33*, 187–205.

Mishra, S. (1992). Leisure activities and life satisfaction in old age: A case study of retired government employees living in urban areas. *Activities and Adaptation, 16*, 7–26.

Mitchell, J. (1975). *The adolescent predicament.* Montreal: Holt, Rinehart and Winston.

Mobily, P., Herr, K., Clark, M., & Wallace, R. (1994). An epidemiologic analysis of pain in the elderly: The Iowa 65+ Rural Health Study. *Journal of Aging and Health, 6*, 139–154.

Mohamed, S., Weisz, G., & Waring, E. (1979). The relationship of chronic pain to depression, marital and family dynamics. *Pain, 5*, 282–292.

Molinari, V. (1991). Mental health issues in the elderly: Strategies and interventions to maintain function. *Physical and Occupational Therapy in Geriatrics, 9*, 23–30.

Moos, R. (1974). *Family Environment Scale: Preliminary manual.* Pale-Alto, CA: Consulting Psychologist Press.

Morley, S. (1993). Vivid memory for "everyday" pains. *Pain, 55*, 55–62.

Mortimer, M., Kay, J., & Jaron, A. (1993). Clinical epidemiology of childhood abdominal migraine in an urban general practice. *Developmental Medicine and Child Neurology, 35*, 243–248.

Mosher, A. (1993). Referral patterns of elderly clients to a community mental health center. *Journal of Gerontological Social Work, 20*, 5–23.

Moskovich, R. (1988). Neck pain in the elderly: Common causes and management. *Geriatrics, 43*, 65–89.

Moss, M., Lawton, M., & Glicksman, A. (1991). The role of pain in the last year of life of older persons. *Journal of Gerontology: Psychological Sciences, 46*, 51–57.

Moss, M., Moss, S., Rubenstein, R., & Resch, N. (1993). Impact of elderly mothers health on middle age daughters. *International Journal of Aging and Human Development, 37*, 1–22.

Muller-Spahn, F., & Hock, C. (1994). Clinical presentation of depression in the elderly. *Gerontology, 40*(Suppl. 1), 10–14.

Murphy, C. (1982). Effects of aging on food perception. *Journal of American College of Nutrition, 1*, 128–133.

Murphy, E. (1982). Social origins of depression. *British Journal of Psychiatry, 141*, 135–142.

MYOPAIN. (1992). Consensus document on fibromyalgia: The Copenhagen declaration. Finalized at the Consensus Conference at the 2nd World Congress on Myofascial Pain and fibromyalgia.

Naidoo, P., & Pillay, Y. (1994). Correlations among general stress, family environment, psychological distress and pain experience. *Perceptual and Motor Skills, 78*, (Special Issue), 1291–1296.

Neugarten, B. (1968). *Middle age and aging: A reader in social psychology.* Chicago: University of Chicago Press.

Nicassio, P., & Radojevic, V. (1993). Models of family functioning and their contribution to patient outcomes in chronic pain. *Motivation and Emotion, 17,* 295–316.

Oen, K., Fast, M., & Postl, B. (1995). Epidemiology of juvenile rheumatoid arthritis in Manitoba, Canada, 1975–1992: Cycles in incidence. *Journal of Rheumatology, 22,* 745–750.

Oles, P. (1994). Construction of a mid-life questionnaire: Assumptions and empirical facts. [Polish] *Przeglad Psychologiczny, 37,* 159–166.

Oppegard, K. (1984). Sensory loss, family support, and adjustment among the elderly. *Journal of Social Psychology, 123,* 291–292.

Pahkala, K. (1990). Social and environmental factors and depression in old age. *International Journal of Geriatric Psychology, 5,* 99–113.

Parmelee, P., Katz, I., & Lawton, M. (1989). Depression among institutionalized aged: Assessment and prevalence estimation. *Journal of Gerontology: Medical Sciences, 44,* M22–M29.

Parmelee, P., Katz, I., & Lawton, M. (1991). The relation of pain to depression among institutionalized aged. *Journal of Gerontology: Psychological Sciences, 46,* P15–P21.

Parmelee, P., Smith, B., & Katz, I. (1993). Pain complaints and cognitive status among elderly institution residents. *Journal of the American Geriatrics Society, 41,* 517–522.

Passchier, J., & Orlebeke, J. F. (1985). Headaches and stress in schoolchildren: An epidemiological study. *Cephalalgia, 5,* 167–176.

Patterson, J. M. (1991). A family systems perspective for working with youth and disability. *Pediatrician, 18*(2), 129–141.

Payne, B., & Norfleet, M. (1986). Chronic pain and the family: A review. *Pain, 26,* 1–22.

Peter, R. (1995). Job stressors, coping characteristics, and the development of coronary heart disease: Results from two studies. [German] *Psychologische Beitrage, 37,* 40–45.

Peterson, C., & Seligman, M. (1984). Causal explanations as a risk factor for depression: Theory and evidence. *Psychological Review, 91,* 347–374.

Peterson, L., Mason, T., Nelson, A., O'Fallon, W., et al. (1996). Juvenile rheumatoid arthritis in Rochester, Minnesota 1960–1993. Is the epidemiology changing. *Arthritis and Rheumatism, 39,* 1385–1390.

Piaget, J., (1972). Intellectual evolution from adolescence to adulthood. *Human Development, 15,* 1–12.

Pilowsky, I., & Bassett, D. (1982). Pain and depression. *British Journal of Psychiatry, 141,* 30–36.

Pina, D., & Bengston, V. (1995). Division of household labor and the well-being of retirement-aged wives. *Gerontologist, 35,* 308–317.

Popescu, V., & Hurduc, V. (1992). Recurrent abdominal pain in children. [Romanian] *Pediatrie, 41,* 50–59.

Potts, M. K., & Silverman, S. L. (1990). The importance of aspects of treatment for fibromyalgia (fibrositis): Differences between patient and physician views. *Arthritis Care and Research, 3*(1), 11–18.

Preston, D., & Dellasega, C. (1990). Elderly women and stress: Does marriage make a difference. *Journal of Gerontological Nursing, 16,* 26–32.

Pribor, E. F., Smith, D. S., & Yutzy, S. H. (1994). Somatization disorder in elderly patients. *American Journal of Geriatric Psychiatry, 2,* 109–117.

Price, D. D., Long, S., & Huitt, C. (1992). Sensory testing of pathophysiological mechanisms of pain in patients with reflex sympathetic dystrophy. *Pain, 49*(2), 163–173.

Procacci, P., Bozza, G., Buzzelli, G., et al. (1970). The cutaneous pain pricking threshold in old age. *Gerontologic Clinics, 12,* 213–218.

Prohaska, T., Leventhal, E., Leventhal, H., & Keller, M. (1985). Health practices and illness cognition in young middle aged and elderly adults. *Journal of Gerontology, 40,* 569–578.

Quirk, M., & Young, M. (1990). The impact of JRA on children, adolescents, and their families: Current research and implications for future studies. *Arthritis Care and Research, 3,* 36–43.

Rangaswami, K. (1983). Stressful life events and neurosis in old age. *Journal of Psychological Research, 27,* 115–119.

Raphael, K., Dohrenwend, B., & Marbach, J. (1990). Illness and injury among children of temporomandibular pain and dysfunction syndrome (TMPDS) patients. *Pain, 40,* 61–64.

Rappaport, L. (1989). Recurrent abdominal pain: Theories and pragmatics. *Pediatrician, 16,* 78–84.

Raspe, H., & Croft, P. (1995). Fibromyalgia. *Bailliere's Clinical Rheumatology, 9,* 599–614.

Raymer, D., Weininger, O., & Hamilton, J. (1984). Psychological problems in children with abdominal pain. *Lancet, 1,* 439–440.

Raymond, B., & Bergland, M. M. (1994). Psychosocial aspects of fibromyalgia syndrome. *Journal of Applied Rehabilitation Counseling, 25*(3), 42–46.

Regier, D., Boyd, J., Burke, J., Jr., Rae, D., Myers, J., et al. (1988). One-month prevalence of mental disorders in the United States. *Archives of General Psychiatry, 45,* 977–986.

Reich, J., Tupin, J., & Abramowitz, S. (1983). Psychiatric diagnosis of chronic pain patients. *American Journal of Psychiatry, 140,* 1495–1498.

Revenson, T., Schiaffino, K., Majerovitz, D., & Gibofsky, A. (1991). Social support as double-edged sword: The relation of positive and problematic support to depression among rheumatoid arthritis patients. *Social Science and Medicine, 33,* 807–813.

Rickard, K. (1988). The occurrence of recurrent maladaptive health-related behaviors and teacher-rated conduct problems in children of chronic low-back pain patients. *Journal of Behavioral Medicine, 11,* 107–116.

Roberts, P., & Newton, P. (1987). Levinsonian studies of women's adult development. *Psychology and Aging, 2,* 154–163.

Robinson, J., Alvarez, J., & Dodge, J. (1990). Life-events and family history in children with recurrent abdominal pain. *Journal of Psychosomatic Research, 34,* 171–181.

Rohling, M., Ellis, N., & Scogin, F. (1991). Automatic and effortful memory processes in elderly persons with organic brain pathology. *Journal of Gerontology, 46,* 137–143.

Romano, J., & Turner, J. (1985). Chronic pain and depression: Does the evidence support a relationship. *Psychology Bulletin, 97,* 18–34.

Romano, J., Turner, J., & Clancy, S. (1989). Sex differences in the relationship of pain patient dysfunction to spouse adjustment. *Pain, 39,* 289–295.

Romano, J., Turner, J., Jensen, M., Friedman, L. et al. (1995). Chronic pain patient–spouse behavioral interactions predict patient disability. *Pain, 63,* 353–360.

Rosenberg, S., & Farrell, M. (1976). Identity and crisis in middle-aged men. *International Journal of Aging and Human Development, 7,* 153–170.

Ross, C., Lavigne, J., Hayford, J., & Berry, S. (1993). Psychological factors affecting reported pain in juvenile rheumatoid arthritis. *Journal of Pediatric Psychology, 18,* 561–573.

Rowat, K., & Knafl, K. (1985). Living with chronic pain: The spouses' perspective. *Pain, 23,* 259–271.

Rowe, J., & Besdine, R. (Eds.). (1982). *Health and disease in old age.* Boston, Little Brown & Co.

Roy, R. (1982). Marital and family issues in patients with chronic pain: A review. *Psychotherapy and Psychosomatics, 37,* 1–12.

Roy, R. (1985). The interactional perspective of pain behavior in marriage. *International Journal of Family Therapy, 7,* 271–283.

Roy, R. (1989). *Family and chronic pain: A systemic perspective.* New York: Human Sciences Press.

Roy, R. (1990). Physical illness, chronic pain and family therapy. In: E. Tunks, A. Bellissimo, & R. Roy (Eds.), *Chronic pain: Psychosocial factors in rehabilitation,* rev. 2nd ed. (pp. 293–000). Malabar, FL: Robert E. Krieger.

Roy, R. (1990–91). Consequences of parental illness on children: A review. *Social Work and Social Science Review, 2,* 109–121.

Roy, R. (1993). Risk factors for suicide among adult alcoholics. *Alcohol, Health and Research World, 17,* 133–136.

Roy, R. (1995). Chronic pain, the elderly and family therapy. In: R. Roy (Ed.), *Chronic pain in old age* (pp. 83–102). Toronto: University of Toronto Press.

Roy, R. (1998). *Child abuse and chronic pain: A curious relationship.* Toronto: University of Toronto Press.

Roy, R., & Frankel, H. (1995). *How good is family therapy? A reassessment.* Toronto: University of Toronto Press.

Roy, R., & Thomas, M. (1986). A survey of chronic pain in an elderly population. *Canadian Family Physicians, 31,* 513–516.

Roy, R., & Thomas, M. (1987). Elderly persons with and without pain. *Clinical Journal of Pain, 3,* 207– 211.

Roy, R., & Thomas, M. (1988). Pain, depression and illness behavior in a group of community based elderly persons: Elderly persons with and without pain. Part II. *Clinical Journal of Pain, 3*(4), 207–211.

Roy, R., & Thomas, M. (1989). Nature of marital relations among chronic pain patients. *Contemporary Family Therapy, 11,* 277–284.

Roy, R., Marykuca, S., Thomas, M., & Cook, A. (1993). In search of pain-prone behavior in a group of college students. *Pain Clinic, 6,* 213–222.

Roy, R., Thomas, M., & Cook, A. (1991). Headache: A family affair. *Headache Quarterly, 2,* 135–137.

Roy, R., Thomas, M., & Cook, A. (1996). University students and their siblings with and without headaches: Comparison of family functioning. Abstracts. 8th World Congress of Pain, International Association for the Study of Pain, Vancouver.

Roy, R., Thomas, M., & Makarenko, P. (1990). A comparative study of pain complaints in a non-clinical Canadian population of university students and seniors. *The Pain Clinic, 3,* 213–222.

Roy, R., Thomas, M., & Matas, M. (1984). Chronic pain and clinical depression: A review. *Comprehensive Psychiatry, 25,* 96–105.

Roy, R., Thomas, M., Mogilevsky, I., & Cook, A. (1994). Influence of parental chronic pain on children. *Headache Quarterly, 5,* 1–7.

Rubenstein, L. Z., & Robbins, A. G. (1984). Falls in the elderly: A clinical perspective. *Geriatrics, 39,* 67–78.

Rubenstein, L. Z., Robbins, A. S., & Josephson, K. P. (1991). Falls in the nursing home setting: Causes and preventive approaches. In: P. R. Katz, R. L. Kane, & M. D. Mezey (Eds.), *Advances in long term care,* Vol. 1 (pp. 28–42). Springer.

Rubin, D. C., & Kozin, M. (1984). Vivid memories. *Cognition, 16*(1), 81–95.

Ruolf, G. (1996). Depression in the patient with chronic pain. *Texas Personnel and Guidance Association Journal, 43,* s25–s34.

Ruskin, P. (1985). Geropsychiatric consultation in a university hospital: A report on 67 referrals. *American Journal of Psychiatry, 142,* 333–336.

Saarijaervi, S. (1991). A controlled study in chronic low back pain patients: Effects on marital satisfaction, psychological distress and health attitudes. *Journal of Psychosomatic Research, 35,* 265–272.

Saarijaervi, S., Hyppae, M. T., Lehtinen, V., & Alanen, E. (1990). Chronic low-back pain patient and spouse. *Journal of Psychosomatic Research, 34,* 117–122.

Salthouse, T. A. (1982). Duration estimates of two information processing components. *Acta Psychologica, 52*(3), 213–226.

Sanders, M., Shepherd, R., Cleghorn, G., & Woodford, H. (1994). The treatment of recurrent abdominal pain in children: A controlled comparison of cognitive–behavioral family intervention and standard pediatric care. *Journal of Consulting Clinical Psychology, 62,* 306–314.

Sartoris, P., & Vanderwell, A. (1981). Student reasons for withdrawing from university of Alberta: 1978–1979. *Canadian Counsellor, 15,* 168–174.

Saxon, S. V. (1991). *Pain management techniques for older adults.* Springfield, IL: Charles C Thomas.

Schoenfeld-Smith, K., Nicassio, P.M, Radojevic, V., & Patterson, T. L. (1995). Multiaxial taxonomy of fibromyalgia syndrome patients. *Journal of Clinical Psychology in Medical Settings, 2*(2), 149–166.

Schon, L., & Zuckerman, J. D. (1988). Hip pain in the elderly: Evaluation and diagnosis. *Geriatrics, 43,* 48–62.

Scott, R. (1994). Recurrent abdominal pain during childhood. *Canadian Family Physician, 40,* 539–542.

Schwartz, L., Slater, M., Birchler, G., & Atkinson, J. (1991). Depression in spouses of chronic pain patients: The role of patient pain, anger, and marital satisfaction. *Pain, 44,* 61–67.

Seip, M. (1994). A study of health status of school children 100 years ago. [Norwegian] *Tidsskr Nor Laegeforen, 114,* 3616–3619.

Sengstaken, E. A., & King, S. A. (1993). The problems of pain and its detection among geriatric nursing home residents. *Journal of the American Geriatrics Society, 41*(5), 541–544.

Shanas, E. (1979). *National survey of the elderly: Report to administration on aging.* Washington, DC: Department of Health and Human Services.

Shanas, E. (1984). Old parents and middle-aged children: The four and five generation family. *Journal of Geriatric Psychiatry, 17,* 7–9.

Shanfield, S., Heiman, E., Cope, N., & Jones, J. (1979). Pain and marital relationship: Psychiatric distress. *Pain, 7,* 24–35.

Siksna, A. (1988). Educational and emotional problems in students in Sweden. *Social Psychiatry and Psychiatric Epidemiology, 23,* 262–263.

Sillanpaa, M. (1976). Prevalence of migraine and other headache in Finnish children starting school. *Headache, 15,* 288–290.

Sillanpaa, M. (1983a). Prevalence of headache in prepuberty. *Headache, 23,* 10–14.

Sillanpaa, M. (1983b). Changes in the prevalence of migraine and other headache during the first seven school years. *Headache, 23,* 15–19.

Simmons, D., & Doherty, W. (1995). Defining who we are and what we do: Clinical practice patterns of marriage and family therapists in Minnesota. *Journal of Marital and Family Therapy, 21,* 3–16.

Skinner, H., Steinhauer, P., & Santa-Barbara, J. (1983). The family assessment measure. *Canadian Journal of Community Mental Health, 2*, 91–105.

Smiley, W., Cram, J., Margoles, Romano, T., & Stiller, J. (1992). Innovations in soft-tissue jurisprudence. *Trial Diplomacy Journal, 15*, 199–208.

Smith, G. (1992). The epidemiology and treatment of depression when it coexists with somatoform disorders, somatization, or pain. Special Section: Developing guidelines for treating depressive disorders in the primary care setting. *General Hospital Psychiatry, 14*, 265–272.

Smith, T., Follick, M., & Ahern, D. (1985). Life-events and psychological disturbance in chronic low-back pain. *British Journal of Clinical Psychology, 24*, 207–208.

Smythe, H., & Moldofsky, H. (1977). Two contributions to understanding of the "fibrositis" syndrome. *Bulletin of Rheumatic Disease, 28*, 928–931.

Sorkin, B., & Turk, D. (1995). Pain management in the elderly. In: R. Roy (Ed.), *Chronic pain in old age: An integrated biopsychosocial perspective* (pp. 137–000). Toronto: University of Toronto Press.

Sorkin, B., Rudy, T., Hanlon, R., Turk, D., & Steig, R. (1990). Chronic pain in old and young patients: Differences appear less important than similarities. *Journal of Gerontology, 45*, 64–68.

Sparks, J. P. (1978). The incidence of migraine in schoolchildren: A survey by the medical officers of schools association. *Practitioner, 221*, 407–411.

Stein, H., Golombek, H., Marton, P., & Korenblum, M. (1991). Consistency and change in personality characteristics and affect from middle to late adolescence. *Canadian Journal of Psychiatry, 36*, 16–19.

Stenager, E. N., Stenager, E., & Jensen, K. (1994). Attempted suicide, depression, and physical diseases: A 1-year follow-up study. *Psychotherapy and Psychosomatics, 61*(1–2), 65–73.

Sternbach, R. (1986a). Survey of pain in the United States: The Nuprin Pain Report. *Clinical Journal of Pain, 2*, 49–53.

Sternbach, R. (1986b). Pain and "hassles" in the United States: Findings of the Nuprin Pain Report. *Pain, 27*, 69–80.

Steven, M. (1992). Prevalence of chronic arthritis in four geographical areas of Scottish Highlands. *Annals of Rheumatic Disease, 51*, 186–194.

Stockton, M., Weinman, J., & McCall, I. (1985). An investigation of psychosocial factors in patients with upper abdominal pain: A comparison with other groups of surgical out-patients. *Journal of Psychosomatic Research, 29*, 191–198.

Stoller, E., & Forster, L. I. (1994). The impact of symptom interpretation of physician utilization. *Journal of Aging and Health, 6*, 507–534.

Sullivan, M., Turner, J., & Romano, J. (1991). Chronic pain in primary care: Identification and management of psychosocial factors. *Journal of Family Practice, 32*, 193–199.

Sweeting, H. (1995). Reversals of fortune: Sex differences in health in childhood and adolescence. *Social Science and Medicine, 40*, 77–90.

Szinovacz, M., & Washo, C. (1992). Gender differences in exposure to life events and adaptation to retirement. *Journal of Gerontology, 47*, s191–s196.

Taal, E., Rasker, J., Seydel, E., & Wiegman, O. (1993). Health status, adherence with health recommendations, self-efficacy and social support in patients with rheumatoid arthritis. *Patient Education and Counselling, 20*, 63–76.

Tansem, L., & Malt, V. F. (1995). Sodium lactate infusion in fibromyalgia patients. *Biological Psychiatry, 38*(8), 559–561.

Teoh, J. (1974). Psychological problems among university students in an area of rapid sociocultural change. *Australian and New Zealand Journal of Psychiatry, 8*, 109–120.

Thomas, M. (1993a). Profiles of pain complaints and psychological functioning in a Canadian university aged population. *VII World Congress on Pain*. Published Abstracts, Paris, France.

Thomas, M. (1993b). Healthy elderly and pain. *Rapport, 1*, 17–18.

Thomas, M. (1994). Comparisons of patterns in reported pain in families between full, half and step siblings. National Council on Family Relations Annual Conference, Minneapolis.

Thomas, M., & Roy, R. (1988a). Age and pain: A comparative study of younger vs. older elderly persons. *Journal of Pain Management Practice, 4*, 174–179.

Thomas, M., & Roy, R. (November 1988b). Variables influencing pain in a Canadian elderly group. Joint Meeting of American and Canadian Pain Societies, Toronto, Ontario.

Thomas, M., & Roy, R. (1989). Pain patients and marital relations. *Clinical Journal of Pain, 5*, 255–259.

Thomas, M., & Roy, R. (1995). Factors from different theoretical perspectives that identify headache in university students. *Headache Quarterly, 6*, 306–312.

Thomas, M., Roy, R., & Cook, A. (1991). Headache, backache, and family for a group of college students and their parents: A follow-up. *Headache Quarterly, 2*, 307–312.

Thomas, M., Roy, R., & Cook, A. (1992). Reports of family pain by college students including a subsample of pain reports of parents. *The Pain Clinic, 5*, 137–145.

Thomas, M., Roy, R., & Makarenko, P. (1989). Social modelling in attitudes toward pain and illness: A comparison of young and elderly subjects. *Journal of Pain Management, 2*, 309–315.

Thomas, M., Roy, R., Cook, A., & Marykuca, S. (1992). Chronic pain in college students: Issues of management. *Canadian Family Physician, 38*, 2597–2601.

Timko, C., Stovel, K., & Baumgartner, M. (1995). Acute and chronic stressors, social resources, and functioning among adolescents with juvenile rheumatic diseases. *Journal of Research on Adolescence, 5*, 361–385.

Timko, C., Stovel, K., & Moos, R. (1992). Functioning among mothers and fathers of children with juvenile rheumatoid arthritis. *Journal of Pediatric Psychology, 17*, 705–724.

Tucker, M., Andrew, M., Ogle, S., & Davison, J. G. (1989). Age-associated change in pain threshold measured by transcutaneous neuronal electrical stimulation. *Age and Aging, 18*, 241–246.

Tulving, E. (1972). Episodic and semantic memory. In: E. Tulving & W. Donaldson (Eds.), *Organization of memory* (pp. 381–403). New York: Academic Press.

Turk, D., Flor, H., & Rudy, T. (1987). Pain and families. I. Etiology, maintenance, and psychosocial impact. *Pain, 30*, 3–27.

Turk, D., Kerns, R., & Rosenberg, R. (1992). Effects of marital interaction on chronic pain and disability: Examining their down-side of social support. *Rehabilitation Psychology, 37*, 259–274.

Turk, D., Okifuji, M., & Scharff, L. (1994). Assessment of older women with chronic pain. In: R. A. Roberts (Ed.), *Older women with chronic pain* (pp. 119–000). New York: Haworth Press.

Turk, D., Okifuji, A., & Scharff, L. (1995). Chronic pain and depression: Role of perceived impact and perceived control in different age cohorts. *Pain, 61*, 93–101.

Turkat, I. (1982). An investigation of parental modeling in the etiology of diabetic illness behavior. *Behavior Research and Theory, 20*, 547–552.

Turkat, I., & Adams, H. (1982). Covert positive reinforcement and pain modification: A test of efficacy and theory. *Journal of Psychosomatic Research, 26*, 191–201.

Turkat, I., Guise, B., & Carter, K. (1983). The effects of vicarious experience on pain termination and work avoidance: Replication. *Behavior Research and Therapy, 21*, 491–493.

Turkat, I., Kuczmierczyk, A., & Adams, H. E. (1984). An investigation of the aetiology of chronic headache: The role of headache models. *Annals of Internal Medicine, 91*, 194–199.

Turnbull, J. (1989). Anxiety and physical illness in the elderly. Symposium: Anxiety: The silent partner (1989, San Francisco, California). *Journal of Clinical Psychiatry, 50*(Suppl.), 40–45.

US Bureau of the Census, International Population Reports. (1992). *An aging world II.* Washington, DC: US Government Printing Office.

Usher, J., & Neisser, U. (1993). Childhood amnesia and the beginnings of memory for four early life events. *Journal of Experimental Psychology: General, 122*, 155–165.

Vaeroy, H. (1996). A contribution to the understanding of pain in fibromyalgia based on cerebrospinal fluid investigations. *Pain Research and Management, 1*, 45–49.

Vahlquist, B. (1955). Migraine in children. *International Archives of Allergy, 7*, 348–355.

Vaillant, G. (1977). *Adaptation to life.* Boston: Little Brown.

Vandvik, I. H. (1990). Mental health and psychosocial functioning in children with recent onset of rheumatic disease. *Journal of Child Psychology and Psychiatry and Applied Disciplines, 31*(6), 961–971.

Vandvik, I., & Forseth, K. (1994). A bio-psychosocial evaluation of ten adolescents with fibromyalgia. *Acta Pediatrica, 83*, 766–771.

Vandvik, I. H., Hoyeraal, H., & Fagurtun, H. (1989). Chronic family difficulties and stressful life-events in recent onset of juvenile arthritis. *Journal of Rheumatology, 16*, 1088–1092.

Varni, J., Wilcox, K., & Hanson, V. (1988). Mediating effects of family social support on child psychological adjustment in juvenile rheumatoid arthritis. *Health Psychology, 7*, 421–431.

Violon, A. (1985). Family etiology of chronic pain. *International Journal of Family Therapy, 7*, 235–246.

Violon, A., & Giurgea, D. (1984). Familial models for chronic pain. *Pain, 18*(2), 199–203.

Virtanen, H. (1993). Family therapy in old age. *Psychiatrica Fennica, 24*, 87–95.

VonKnorring, L., Perris, C., Eisemann, M., Eriksson, U., & Perris, H. (1983). Pain as a symptom in depressive disorders. I. Relationship to diagnostic subgroup and depressive symptomatology. *Pain, 15*, 19–26.

Von Korff, M. (1992). Epidemiologic and survey methods: Chronic pain assessment. In: D. C. Turk & R. Melzack (Eds.), *Handbook of pain assessment* (pp. 391–408). New York: Guilford.

Von Korff, M., & Simon, G. (1996). The relationship between pain and depression. *British Journal of Psychiatry, 168*(Suppl. 30), 101–108.

Von Korff, M., Dworkin, S. F., leResche, L., & Kruger, A. (1988). An epidemiological comparison of pain complaints. *Pain, 32*(2), 173–183.

Waddell, G. (1987). A new clinical model for the treatment of low-back pain. *Spine, 12*, 632–644.

Walker, L., & Zemen, J. (1992). Parental response to child illness behavior. *Journal of Pediatric Psychology, 17*, 49–71.

Walker, L., Garber, J., & Greene, J. (1993). Psychosocial correlates of recurrent childhood pain: A comparison of pediatric patients with recurrent abdominal pain, organic illness, and psychiatric disorders. *Journal of Abnormal Psychology, 102*, 248–258.

Walker, L., Garber, G., & Greene, J. (1994). Somatic complaints in pediatric patients: A prospective study of the role of negative life events, child social and academic competence, and parental somatic symptoms. *Journal of Consulting Clinical Psychology, 62*, 1213–1221.

Wall, P. D. (1990). *Altered sensation and pain.* Basel, Switzerland: S. Karger AG, viii, 212 pp.

Wallander, J., & Varni, W. (1989). Social support and adjustment in chronically ill and handicapped children. *American Journal of Community Psychology, 17*, 185–201.

Wampler, R., Fischer, J., Thomas, M., & Lyness, K. (1993). Young adult offspring and their families of origin: Cohesion, adaptability and addiction. *Journal of Substance Abuse, 5*, 195–201.

Waskell, S., & Owens, R. (1991). Frequency distribution of trigger events identified by people aged 30 through 60. *College Student Journal, 25*, 235–239.

Waters, W. E. (1970). Community studies of the prevalence of headache. *Headache, 9*, 178–186.

Weickgenant, A. L., Slater, M., & Patterson, T. (1993). Coping activities in chronic low-back pain: Relationship with depression. *Pain, 53*, 95–103.

Weinberg, H., Wadsworth, J., & Baron, R. (1983). Demand and the impact of leading questions on eyewitness testimony. *Memory and Cognition, 11*, 101–104.

Weinberger, M., Hiner, S., & Tierney, W. (1987). Assessing social support in elderly adults. *Social Science and Medicine, 25*, 1049–1055.

Weinberger, M., Tierney, W., Boober, P., & Hiner, S. (1990). Social support, stress and functional status in patients with osteoarthritis. *Social Science and Medicine, 30*, 503–508.

Weir, R., Browne, G., Tunks, E., & Gafni, A. (1992). A profile of users of specialty pain clinic services: Predictors of use and cost estimates. *Journal of Clinical Epidemiology, 45*, 1399–1415.

Weller, E. B., & Weller, R. A. (Eds.). *Current perspectives on major depressive disorders in children.* Washington, DC: American Psychiatric Press.

Wheatley, D. (1988). Use of anti-anxiety drugs in the medically ill. *Psychotherapy and Psychosomatics, 49*, 63–80.

Williamson, G., & Schulz, R. (1992). Pain, activity restriction, and symptoms of depression among community-residing elderly adults. *Journal of Gerontology, 47*, 367–372.

Williamson, G., & Schulz, R. (1995). Activity restriction mediates the association between pain and depressed affect: A study of younger and older adult cancer patients. *Psychology and Aging, 10*, 369–378.

Wolf, B. (1978). behavioral measures of human pain. *The Psychology of Pain, 20*, 129–168.

Wolfe, F., Ross, K., Anderson, J., Russell, I. J., & Hebert, L. (1995). The prevalence and characteristics of fibromyalgia in the general population. *Arthritis and Rheumatism, 38*, 19–28.

Wolfe, F., Smythe, H., Yunus, M., Bennett, R., et al. (1990). The American College of

Rheumatology 1990 criteria for the classification of fibromyalgia: Report of the multicenter criteria committee. *Arthritis and Rheumatism, 33,* 160–172.
Woo, J., Ho, S., Lau, J., Yuen, Y., et al. (1994). *Acta Psychiatrica Scandinavica, 89,* 8–13.
Woods, R. (1993). Psychosocial management of depression. *International Review of Psychiatry, 5,* 427–436.
Wright, L., & Moore, R. (1982). Correlations of reported drug abuse problems among college undergraduates. *Journal of Drug Education, 12,* 65–73.
Yagill, D. (1991). Self-concept and perceived change among women in their thirties. *Israel Journal of Psychology, 2,* 139–149.
Zauta, A., Marbach, J. J., & Raphael, K. (1995). The examination of myofascial pain and its relationship to psychological distress in women. *Health Psychology, 14,* 223–231.
Ziesat, H. A. (1978). Are family patterns related to the development of chronic low back pain? *Perceptual and Motor Skills, 46*(3, pt. 2), 1062–0000.
Zuckerman, B., Stevenson, J., & Bailey, V. (1987). Stomachaches and headaches in a community samples of preschool children. *Pediatrics, 79,* 677–682.

Index